FROM LORI & ROBIN FOR CHRISTMAS '85
MAY 23, 1986

FROM LORI & ROBIN FOR CHRISTMAS '85
MAY 23, 1986

The Businessman's Minutes-a-Day Guide to Shaping Up

The Businessman's Minutes-a-Day Guide to Shaping Up

Dr. Franco Columbu

WITH LYDIA FRAGOMENI

Contemporary Books, Inc.
Chicago

Library of Congress Cataloging in Publication Data

Columbu, Franco.
 The businessman's minutes-a-day guide to shaping up.

 Includes index.
 1. Men—Health and hygiene.   2. Businessmen—
Nutrition.   3. Exercise.   4. Physical fitness.
I. Title.
RA777.8.C64   1983   613.7′044   83-7747
ISBN 0-8092-5580-4

Exercise photos by Robert Gardner.

Drawings by D. Drake.

Copyright © 1983 by Franco Columbu
All rights reserved
Published by Contemporary Books, Inc.
180 North Michigan Avenue, Chicago, Illinois 60601
Manufactured in the United States of America
Library of Congress Catalog Card Number: 83-7747
International Standard Book Number: 0-8092-5580-4 (cloth)

Published simultaneously in Canada by
Beaverbooks, Ltd.
195 Allstate Parkway
Valleywood Business Park
Markham, Ontario L3R 4T8
Canada

Contents

Introduction

Never have so many people taken into their own hands the responsibility for getting fit and staying fit. At present more than 70 million adults are doing some type of exercise daily, which is more than double the number who were exercising in 1960 and triple the number in 1940. For every person you see jogging down the street, another 90 are doing some form of exercise, from bicycling to cross-country skiing. More than 25 million train with weights either to get into shape or to improve their performance in other sports.

This exercise boom was triggered in the 1950s by a study revealing that the fitness level of American children was far below the level of children in Switzerland, Austria, and Italy. Concerned by this report, President Eisenhower established the Council on Youth Fitness in 1956, which later enlarged its focus and became the President's Council on Physical Fitness and Sport.

Since these early days the word *fitness* has fallen on our ears a thousand times, being defined many different ways. To some men, being fit means little more than losing 10 pounds, hopefully around the waist and abdominal area, where it is highly visible not only to themselves but to everyone else. To other men, it means having the stamina to get through a day's work with enough energy left over to enjoy leisure activities or to take classes toward an academic degree. Others measure fitness by the distance they run, the strength of their tennis stroke, or the ability to mow a lawn or drive long distances without suffering from a stiff back.

Appearance

There was a time when a man's prosperity was measured by the size of his potbelly. Often excess poundage dignified certain individuals as thinkers, too busy using their brains to indulge time on appearance. However, the portly men who once dominated business and industry are gradually being replaced by others who have a keen awareness of the benefits derived from maintaining a vigorous physical appearance.

Today a man's ability to perform well on the job is quite often determined by giving the impression of being strong and powerful. The complexity of business has increased tenfold during the past 25 years, demanding highly integrated individuals who can attend to the many different facets of running an organization. A well-molded and maintained physique seems to reflect the inner strength to cope with pressure, formidable obstacles, fragmentation, and other stresses that accompany high-level positions.

Recently a study was done by several major corporations whose executives were on specific exercise training programs. The findings showed that strict adherence to the programs increased the executive's aggressiveness, performance level, and ability to handle stress. In addition, they received a boost to their egos when secretaries and other women on the office staff began complimenting them on their appearance.

Of course, it is a pleasure to look terrific and know that your clothes fit well, but even more valuable is the realization of having greatly reduced tendencies toward hypertension, so you can be more aggressive with less stress. By increasing circulation throughout your body you can acquire greater virility and a dynamic sex life. Training regularly also produces the advantage of sweating less during business meetings. When you are obviously cool and collected others receive the positive impression that you have everything under control.

Often it is said, "One picture is worth a thousand words," and this goes for your personal appearance throughout the day and all the years of your life.

This book is directed toward reaching all these goals and even more, since physical fitness is made up of many components, including a well-proportioned body, muscular strength and endurance, flexibility, cardiorespiratory efficiency, and good nutrition. I have considered all these factors in designing the best bodybuilding programs to get you into shape without wasted effort in minimal time. Equally important are the maintenance programs developed to keep you in shape once you have done the hard work of reaching your goals.

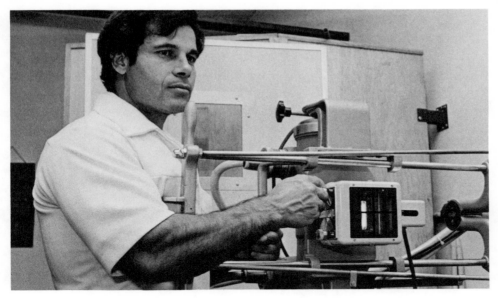

Dr. Columbu has been in chiropractic practice for over 15 years. His background in kinesiology, physiology, and nutrition has helped him develop a physique admired by thousands of bodybuilding fans.

You will have a selection of routines from which to choose—whether you work out at home, in a gym, or on the road—as well as exercises that can easily be done in your office. I have provided detailed information on equipment needed to accommodate every budget along with recommendations for choosing a gym, home exercise units, nutrition, and losing weight without suffering from highly restrictive diets. Because I receive countless letters and phone calls from people around the world asking for advice on injuries, I have included a section on causes, prevention, and treatment of injuries.

More than a dozen specialized programs were developed for those wanting to improve performance in other sports, since weight training increases the muscle strength and endurance needed for balance, agility, and stamina. In conjunction with this are exercises for improving the game of your choice. For instance, while playing tennis you can get your hips, thighs, and stomach into shape with little additional effort.

The programs that follow will deliver exactly what they promise. I created them by studying the way my own body successfully responded to different training routines and by observing the progress made by thousands who have come to the Columbu Chiropractic Center for consultation and treatment. Among my clients are men of all ages: celebrities, sports figures, and those in every occupation, from mechanics to computer programmers to top level executives. They share with you the need to improve themselves by keeping in shape to reap the benefits of their full potential. It was highly gratifying to see them reach the goals they set. I have written this book with the expectation of guiding you along the same successful road.

One

Richard Newcombe: A Record of Goal Setting and Accomplishment

Very often people say, "I've lost 10 or 20 pounds, but I still feel fat." This was the case with Rick Newcombe, one of my students, when he first came to see me at the Chiropractic Center.

Rick is vice-president and general manager of the Los Angeles Times Syndicate, a division of the *Los Angeles Times* that sells columns, cartoons, comic strips and book serializations to newspapers across the country and around the world. He is now 32 years old and lives in Santa Monica, California, with his wife and two small children.

At the time of his first visit to my office Rick had lost 20 pounds by going to Weight Watchers meetings and following their diet program. He was running two miles a day and had been working out in a gym for approximately two months. Despite this, the skin around his waist and chest was flabby from the weight loss, and he still had fat deposits that hadn't burned off. The muscular, rock-hard look he wanted to achieve seemed unattainable

After a consultation I gave him a bodybuilding program that enabled him to reach his goals in about a year. During this time he kept a training diary to plan time for his workouts, set goals, and record progress. Because Rick's story is typical of what can be accomplished by the average businessman wanting to get into top shape, I asked him to share the record of his experience and success in following one of my shape-up programs. His story follows.

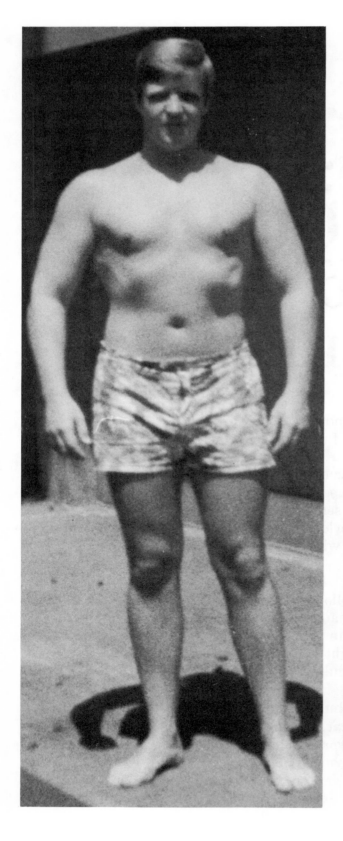 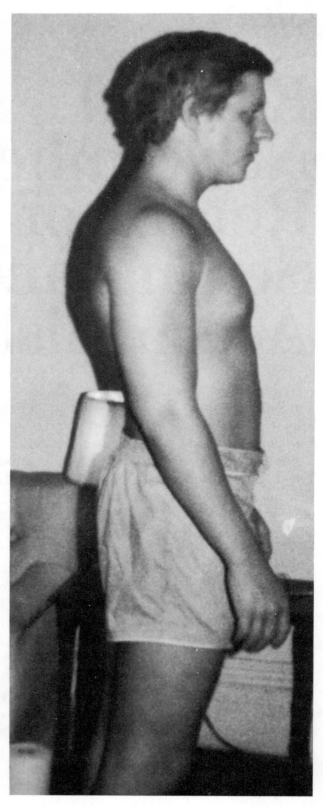

January 1981: Facing Hard Facts

The history of my losing weight and gaining muscle on a bodybuilding program starts in January 1981, when I weighed 191 pounds. At 5'10" I was carrying at least 30 pounds of excess weight, most of it fat. All my shirt collars felt too tight and my pants were tight around the waist and thighs. Each time I put my belt on and slipped the buckle into the last notch I faced the hard fact that the next belt I bought would be a size 38. Now I weigh 154 pounds and my belt size is 30. I take great enjoyment in having people at work tell me how great I look in a suit. But back in January 1981 I was desperate to lose the excess weight I had begun accumulating at the rate of five pounds a year since the age of 24. The gain had been gradual enough but had ended up being 30 pounds of pure fat.

In January of 1981 I joined Weight Watchers, going on their diet program and attending the weekly meetings until May. About the same time I decided to take up running. I began by walking one mile a day and gradually worked up to running half a mile by concentrating on running as slowly as possible. There were times in those early days of running in the park that people walking fast actually passed me, but I didn't care. I kept at it, and by May of 1981 I was able to run two miles a day. I looked a lot better, having lost about 20 pounds by going to Weight Watchers, but the skin around my waist and chest was flabby from the weight loss and because I still had a lot of body fat.

June 1981: Joining a Gym

In June of 1981 I decided to join a gym and combine weight training with running. It wouldn't be the first time in my life that I had lifted a barbell. At the age of 13 I had a goal of becoming Mr. America, a goal that is probably the dream of a great many teenage boys. Because it was really important to me I did more than dream about reaching my goal. At the time I lived in Chicago, and every Saturday I went to a health food store in the downtown area to see a man called Rock Stonewall—I believe his first name was really Jesse, but everyone called him Rock. He was my hero, and building as much muscle as Rock became my next goal. Although he gave me a great deal of good advice, I never stuck with it, instead becoming involved in regular sports such as soccer and swimming. While in college I signed up for a membership at a health spa but dropped out after a short time. In 1978, while living on the East Coast, I joined a Holiday Health Club. After working out casually for a couple of months, however, I never went back. Later I was to discover that I could stick with my training program developed by Franco because I returned to his office every few months to report on my progress.

But in June 1981 I was still on my own, trying to find the best way to build muscle and get myself into top shape. This time I signed up for a 90-day program at Gold's Gym in Venice, California, and began lifting weights from two to four times a week. I also bought a number of fitness magazines and weight training courses. It didn't take long to discover that there were as many different opinions on weight training as there were bodybuilders. For instance, one bodybuilder advised doing only one or two sets of exercises per body part. Another stated that the only way to make significant gains was by working out three to four hours a day, six days a week. A third firmly held the opinion that Nautilus, Universal Gym, and other machines were the only way to go. In direct opposition, another said that free weights were the best equipment to use. Some gave orders to exercise very strictly with full movements while others gave permission to cheat by swinging the weights.

I experimented with all these different programs for a couple of months, finally deciding that this method of trial and error was a mistake at my age. I was a 31-year-old executive with a highly responsible job and a family, not a teenage boy with plenty of gym time to experiment. My career is very important to me and I am extremely close to my wife and children, so my free time was already in great demand. There was no room to reinvent the wheel, especially if I could get advice from a professional who had devoted the better part of his life to the study and understanding of physiology, exercise, and nutrition.

From reading fitness magazines and working out in a gym I had come to know about many experts. After making a list of their names and looking it over, I decided the best one was Franco Columbu. He was a doctor of chiropractic with a PhD in nutrition, but even more important, he was Mr. Olympia and had obviously developed a huge amount of muscle. I liked the way he looked—rock-hard without fat. Whenever you see a picture of Franco Columbu he never seems fat: always he maintains that strong, chiseled look.

July 30, 1981: An Appointment with Franco

My next step was to call the Columbu Chiropractic Center in Westwood, California, to ask if Franco's practice also included designing training programs for bodybuilding. Being told that it did, I made an appointment to see him on July 30, 1981. My decision to see Franco followed the same logic as studying with the best piano

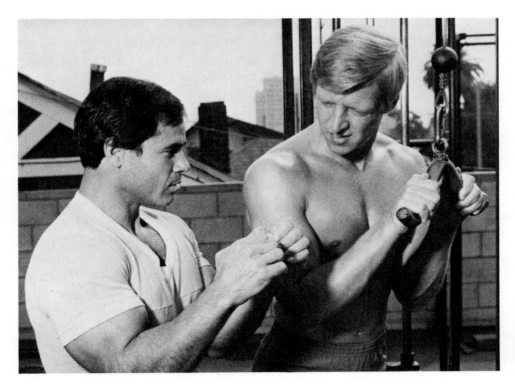

Franco demonstrates how to grip handle of pulley for Pulley Pushdown exercise.

teacher if I wanted to play the piano well or taking speed reading classes to improve my reading skills or skiing lessons if I wanted to become a skier.

At my first meeting with Franco I told him about my gains and improvements that had resulted from the Weight Watchers program and from running two miles a day. I explained my frustration at still having a lot of fat on my body and being unable to develop a rock-hard look.

Even before Franco opened his mouth I had decided to follow his advice no matter what he said. I was more than ready. Days of trial, error, and confusion, caused by a multitude of conflicting opinions, were over and I was anxious to place myself in the hands of the expert I had so carefully chosen. Since that first visit with Franco many men have approached me in the gym and offered advice, but I have consistently checked it out with Franco before taking any of it seriously. From that first day he has been the final authority for me.

This unwavering trust has allowed me to avoid grappling with any doubts concerning my training program. The experience is similar to being in college and accepting the fact that certain courses are needed to meet graduation requirements. In the same way I have followed Franco's advice and profited from the peace of mind that comes from not looking at too many alternatives, knowing that I am on the right track.

My decision to follow Franco's advice exclusively was reinforced at a recent business luncheon with Arnold Schwarzenegger. We met to discuss business connected with some of his books that had been syndicated as newspaper serializations. When I spoke of my decision to go with Franco no matter what, Arnold replied that I had made the smartest possible move. He said that Franco knew more about the human body and muscle building than anyone else, not only from his own experience but also as a result of his studies and research. "And in addition," said Arnold, "it makes good sense not to go through trial and error in the 1980s when a successful bodybuilding program is no longer a big mystery." He felt Franco's knowledge was superior for training others to shape their bodies whether they wanted to gain or lose weight or build muscle.

In almost every respect Arnold's feelings were similar to my own when I decided to see Franco in July of 1981. It was during this first visit that I showed Franco some of my pictures. While it seemed I had lost a great deal of weight and made significant progress, he looked at the pictures and pointed out fat deposits on my face and around my chest, waist, and buttocks.

Franco said, "The best way to burn off fat is by exercising fairly rapidly with weights and doing a high number of repetitions for body parts needing the most work. For you, Rick, it's better to work up a sweat by going rapidly rather than using heavy weights and exercising slowly."

He wanted me to begin by focusing on particular areas, not only to get into shape but also to balance my body. Franco advised continuing a Weight Watchers type of program and gave me a balanced diet with recommendations to cut down on milk, yogurt, and cream in my coffee, since dairy products caused the formation of fat beneath the skin.

When I looked at the weight training routine Franco designed for me I thought the number of sets and repetitions was next to impossible. However, directly after our meeting I went to Gold's Gym and started working out. About halfway through the session I got a headache that was so bad it was necessary to stop training and go home and take some aspirin. I began experiencing doubt concerning my commitment to a demanding weight training program. Bodybuilding and business didn't seem very compatible. I was troubled by the thought that business responsibilities should be my prime concern and not working out in a gym. I kept asking myself, "What am I doing with all this serious training?" On this doubtful note I ended the first day of trying to adjust to the initial training program.

To my surprise I awoke the following morning feeling so refreshed that I returned to the gym and trained very hard. At some point I began feeling incredibly exhilarated, as if I had plugged into some vast new source of energy from within. Perhaps working out early in the morning had something to do with it. I still prefer beginning my workout at 6:00 in the morning and watching the sun come up as I lift and lower weights. Then, when I finish at 7:30 or 8:00, it feels as if I'm starting the day right by getting my blood circulating. After taking a shower and having a big breakfast I head downtown to my office at the Los Angeles Times Syndicate, always feeling as if I can conquer the world. Although a full day of work with all of its major concerns and responsibilities is still ahead, I never wonder about having the stamina to confront it.

Initial Program

The basic program Franco outlined in the summer of 1981 was a split routine requiring me to train four days a week. A *split routine* is a way of training particular body parts during one training session, leaving other parts to be trained during another session. In this way, I could concentrate all my effort on one or two groups of muscles instead of the whole body. The following list was how Franco suggested I "split" my body:

> Chest, shoulders, and back: twice a week
> Arms and legs: twice a week
> Calves: three or four times a week
> Stomach: each session

Franco prescribed the following list of exercises, sets, and repetitions (reps) for each of my muscle groups. The way the "prescription" is presented in a bodybuilder's shorthand: the exercise name followed by two numbers separated by a multiplication sign. For example, "Bench Press 4 × 12" means doing a total of 48 bench presses in 4 *sets* of 12 *reps*. The first set of 12 reps should be a warm-up set with light weights (if not just the barbell bar!), a rest interval of a minute or less, another set of 12 reps with a heavier weight, rest, and so on with progressively heavier poundages added to the barbell.

(Suggestions for beginning poundages will be provided in Chapter 3.)

Chest Exercises

Bench Press (40 lbs)	4 × 12
Incline Bench Press (30 lbs)	4 × 12
Dips	2 × 10
Pullover (20 lbs)	2 × 10

Shoulder Exercises

Press behind Neck (30 lbs)	3 × 12
Bent-Over Lateral Raise (10 lbs ea)	4 × 12
Standing Lateral Raise (10 lbs ea)	4 × 10
Front Raise (10 lbs ea)	2 × 10

Back Exercises

Chins	3 × 5
Pulldown (70 lbs)	5 × 10
One-Arm Rowing (20 lbs)	2 × 10
Barbell Rowing (40 lbs)	4 × 10

Arm Exercises

Triceps Pulldown (40 lbs)	4 × 12
Seated Dumbbell Curl on Incline Bench (20 lbs ea)	3 × 10
Triceps Press, Lying on Back (30 lbs)	4 × 10
Preacher Curl (20 lbs ea)	3 × 10

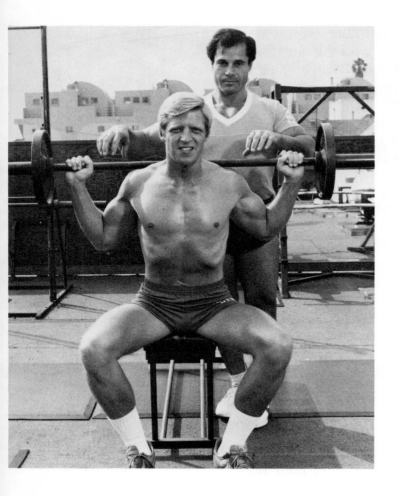

Leg Exercises

Squats (60 lbs ea)	3 × 15
Leg Extension (20 lbs)	5 × 25
Leg Curl (20 lbs)	2 × 25
Calf Raise (100 lbs)	5 × 15

Stomach Exercises

Crunch	1 × 25
Bent-Leg Sit-Up	1 × 25
Side Leg Raise	1 × 25
Side Bend	1 × 25

Another important part of my shape-up program is running. Franco suggested that I run four times a week to maintain aerobic fitness, but not more than two miles. According to his research when you run more than 2 miles a day over an extended period, the body adapts by making the upper body thin out while making the legs bigger. I have continued the same basic routine since my first meeting with Dr. Columbu. In this way I know my heart stays in good shape while I build muscle strength and endurance with weight training.

Working Out

When I first started training I was extremely self-conscious, and like most guys at the gym, I exercised mechanically without ever going all out. Again it was Franco's advice that helped. "You've got to lose yourself at the gym," he said. "Start working like crazy to make your muscles blow up like balloons and forget the other guys. Think only about the workout and building your muscles." At the next session in the gym I started making noises while exercising, grunting and groaning and at times shouting, without caring if this bothered others or if they laughed at the funny faces I was making. As Franco had told me, by concentrating on building muscle and losing myself in the workout I was able to channel my energy into a positive force that blotted out all feelings of self-consciousness.

Trying to adjust to the initial training routine, I experienced several other problems. For instance, I was getting a kink in my neck which I later discovered came from doing side laterals. While doing them I kept jerking my head up instead of keeping it straight by focusing my eyes on a corner of the room between the floor and the wall. Also, I didn't follow the routine Franco had outlined for chest exercises. Using only light dumbbells, I did only two sets of bench presses and perhaps two sets of dips. Part of my reason was the inability to do more than five dips in a row. Today I find this mind-boggling since I can do 35 dips, even finding it necessary to use weights for added resistance.

At the time, however, I was concerned about getting a fat chest since I had fat deposits around my nipples. Franco said, "It's impossible; fat only accumulates more on body parts not exercised. Any area regularly trained becomes muscular." With this in mind I flipped through a fitness magazine and looked at pictures of female body-builders. Seeing that none had full breasts, I figured they worked off fat by exercising their chests. Today I'm training hard to make up for five or six months of not doing the number of chest exercises originally outlined by Franco.

A year ago I found it impossible to do more than one wide-grip chin without resting. I thought of cheating, that is, using only the negative resistance of lowering my body and using a chair to jump back to the top position. Franco disagreed, saying it was better to do one complete rep, rest, do another, and then rest again. Today I can do 10 wide-grip chins, having worked hard to develop the strength and muscle endurance of the latissimus dorsi.

September 1981

On September 6, 1981, I made a notation in my training diary not to miss a single workout during the month. Keeping this diary had become important not only to record goals but also to plan time for working out, resting, and laying off (not training for one week every two or three months). Other than planned layoffs, I continue working out four days a week: Sunday, Monday, Wednesday, and Saturday mornings. If I can't train on one of these days, I make it up during the same week on another day.

On September 27 the notation in my diary read, "Goals reached!" Listing short-term goals served as a driving force and gave me a sense of accomplishment. Upon successfully reaching one goal I set another, bringing me closer to attaining the rock-hard look that was my final aim. This time I was particularly pleased to go through the entire month without missing a training session. Now the thought of skipping a workout never occurs to me. There's nothing like getting that pump and feeling the warm blood coming through, nourishing and enlarging the muscles in my arms, chest, back, and shoulders. As Franco has said, "Work like crazy to make your muscles blow up like balloons."

During this period of time my membership at Gold's Gym ran out, so I switched to World Gym in Santa Monica. It was a good move, despite my feelings of embarrassment in the beginning when I was using light weights and many of the other guys were lifting much heavier ones. However, I learned not to let this bother me, taking a similar path to that of running slowly when I first started a fitness program. Overcoming self-consciousness in any new endeavor is based on ignoring others who are more experienced and focusing only on yourself and your goals. Now I am as strong as many of the guys who were lifting heavier weights, and by continuing to work hard I become stronger at each training session.

I rate World Gym as one of the best for serious training because it is extremely well equipped and well organized. Five different sets of dumbbells, ranging in weight from 15 to 60 pounds, are always set into racks where they belong when not in use. This eliminates time spent hunting around the gym and under equipment for the missing mate of a dumbbell. Also available are three bars for dips, three squat racks, and so much additional machinery that I have never stood around waiting for three other guys to finish using a piece of equipment. In this way I am spared the disadvantage of having my warmed-up muscles cool off between sets of exercises.

My experience in training in a number of different gyms around the country when on business trips has shown me that most other gyms fall short of the standards established by Joe Gold, owner of World Gym. Approximately every two months I travel to the East Coast or to big cities in the Midwest like Chicago and Detroit. After checking into the hotel I always look up a gym so my schedule of training can continue without interruption. I am continually amazed to find many gyms on the East Coast set up like dungeons in the basements of buildings and gyms that resemble junk shops where it is impossible to find a set of 30-pound dumbbells. Many times I found only one 20- and one 30-pound dumbbell, making me wonder how members of those gyms train without becoming strangely lopsided. In some places the weights were so loosely socketed that they shook and wobbled as I did pullovers, making me guard against the weight dropping off and smashing my teeth.

October 29–Christmas 1981

When I saw Franco in October of 1981 he said that I was much improved, having lost a lot of fat and gained muscle. His encourage-

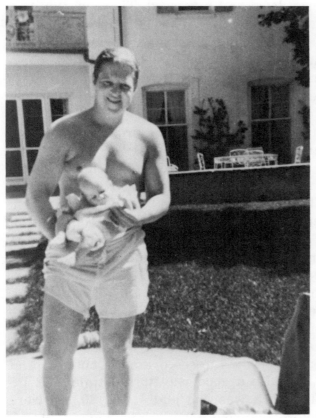 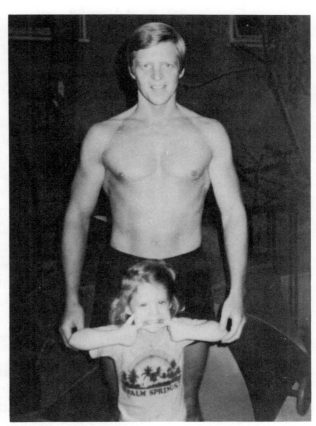

The ultimate comparison photo—a little more than three years of exercise yields ten years in youthful appearance.

ment kept me going more than I can say. I asked him about the "sticking points" that everyone was always warning me about, saying that the first few months were easy but afterward all gains came to a dead stop. "Nonsense," Franco answered. "Just stick with the program. You can increase the number of sets a little by doing four instead of three for some of the weaker body parts. Meanwhile, don't listen to anyone with negative opinions; they can only drag you down. Concentrate on the training program, and by Christmas you'll show even greater improvement." That was my goal, to look better by Christmas, so I stuck with it, increasing the number of sets for some exercises such as those for my shoulders, which have always been my weakest part and required hard training. Being able to see Franco and get the benefit of his advice and encouragement was like having an outside mirror reflecting my ultimate aim.

Around the middle of December I had some pictures taken that showed the improvement Franco had predicted. Comparing these photographs with others taken before starting the program Franco had outlined, I saw a good measure of improvement in the amount of fat lost and muscle gained. With this significant progress toward my goal I found that my energy level had increased. There was quite a change from those days when I was feeling fat and flabby, consuming more calories than I could burn off dieting and running. Back then I skipped breakfast, ate a big lunch, and usually had a few drinks before dinner. This pattern of eating, fairly typical among businessmen, leads to feeling sluggish in the morning and tired in the afternoon. Today my diet is balanced, consisting of low-fat foods, fruits, and salads that, in addition to the training program, make me feel light and energetic all the time.

At Christmas of 1981 I went to Chicago to see my folks. It was quite a celebration, with my seven brothers and sisters and their spouses flying in from all parts of the country for a family reunion. Adding to the good cheer and festivity was my family commenting on the obvious amount of muscle I had developed. My brother Ray, a doctor and marathon runner, was particularly encouraging, saying that I was adding years to my life by getting into top shape.

Also, whenever in Chicago I train with an old friend, Paul Wing. Seeing Paul once or twice a year gives us an excellent opportunity to compare our measures of progress, since lasting gains come gradually and are difficult to observe on a daily basis. The perspective of time between our workouts allows us to see dramatic changes and improvements. Children are also a good way to tell time. For instance, when my daughter Sara was one and I was 30, we were photographed together before I started getting into shape. Pictures taken today, when she is 3 and I am 32, show us *both* looking totally different. Although my son Jack is still a baby, the pleasure of watching him grow has given me a good incentive to change along with him as we develop ourselves in separate ways.

January 2, 1982

Returning to see Franco on January 2, 1982, I showed him a fitness magazine with the photographs of a sportscaster who had developed a lot of muscle.

"How long would it take me to look like him?" I asked Franco.

"In August you'll look like him," he said.

I was taken aback by his answer. According to the magazine article, it took five years of training for the sportscaster to achieve his muscularity. Yet looking at my pictures taken in August, eight months after Franco's prediction, it was evident that he was right. Not only had I developed as much muscle as the sportscaster, I looked even better.

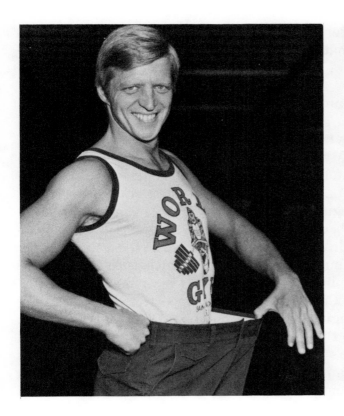
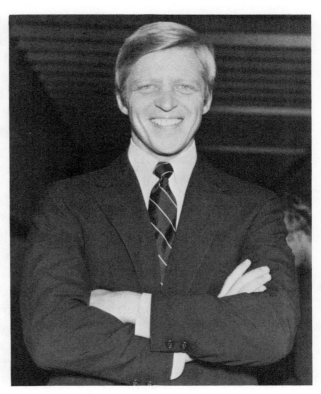

April 1982

During the spring and summer of 1982 my rate of progress took a great leap forward that can be attributed chiefly to the power of visualization. I bought movies of Franco training and had them transferred to tapes for my videocassette player. Watching them as well as the movie *Pumping Iron* as much as possible made my workouts easier. Looking at the films gave me the ability to visualize the workout before actually going to the gym and training. It became a matter of seeing how I wanted to look as a movie in my mind. The power of this repeated visualization was incredible, and the enormous improvement it effected was obvious when I compared my photographs taken before and after the spring of '82

In April, when spending a few days in Palm Springs, I received some complimentary feedback that was totally unexpected. One morning I got up early to run before the desert heat set in. After running two miles I walked another two because walking burns off fat without taking away muscle size. By this time it had become quite hot, so I pulled off my tank top, which left me wearing only my shorts and running shoes. Walking briskly just ahead of me was an older woman who was extremely trim and fit. As I passed by she looked at me and said, "Young man, you look fantastic!" Her compliment made me feel terrific, since it seemed to come from her so naturally. I'll admit that she caught me off guard a little because no one, particularly not a perfect stranger, had ever said anything similar.

As I continued walking I couldn't help looking at my reflection in the store windows. She's right, I thought; I do look fantastic. There was a real glow to my skin and virtually no fat on my body, just a great deal of muscle. My tan enhanced the total look of a man in top physical condition. Later that morning I went to the pool and swam about a dozen laps. An attractive woman who was sitting by the pool kept watching me (I guess this was my day for being admired by women). When I climbed out of the pool she asked if I was a college football player. I couldn't get over it. Here I was, an executive in my 30s with such a good build that she believed I was a college football player. It is little compliments like these that really keep you going.

Of course, my wife Carole was highly supportive of my training program from the beginning. Since I taped all my sessions with Franco, Carole listened to the tapes when I brought them home and was struck by Franco's intelligence and sensible advice. Carole has begun her own program of swimming or jogging for 30 minutes a day, attributing her enthusiasm for this exercise to my example. Friends have commented that she is trimmer and more vibrant today than five years ago before our children were born.

The Power of Goal Setting

Around the middle of April I went to New York on business. While sitting alone in my hotel room I read a book that stated that the key to successful goal setting lies in having an exact mental picture of the wanted result and setting a deadline for achieving it. Since it was April 17, I set my goal six months ahead to October 17, planning to have my picture taken while wearing workout trunks or a bathing suit. I would pose either flexing my muscles or standing relaxed, or perhaps doing both. As the book on goal setting had suggested, I had an exact mental picture of the way I wanted to look by October 17.

October 17, 1982

As a dry run in August, I had some pictures taken by a friend that look very good, particularly when compared with others taken one year before. After seeing them, Franco asked if I would be interested in writing about my weight training experience for a chapter in his next book. He also wanted to know if I would pose for some pictures of exercises illustrating the text.

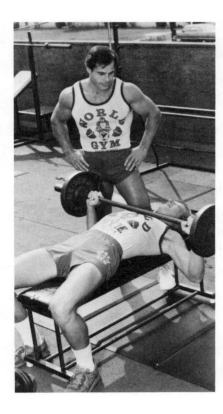
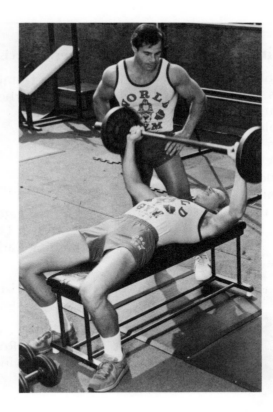

Franco supervises as Richard Newcombe performs Barbell Bench Presses.

"When are you taking the pictures?" I asked. When he said that they would be taken in October it amazed me since I had set my big goal for that exact period of time. To me this reinforced the power of goal setting, which like a magnet drew me into writing this chapter. After all, Franco was not aware of my goal for October, and I didn't know he was writing another book due for production in the fall.

It has really boosted my ego to have Franco ask me to write about my record of goal setting and accomplishment for the benefit of others. Only two years ago I was a typical overweight businessman who was eating too much red meat and white bread with butter, gobbling peanuts, snacking on pizza and potato chips, drinking beer and scotch at night and milk during the day, and adding a generous measure of cream and sugar to my coffee. If dessert was offered after lunch, I readily accepted it, and while traveling on the road for business I ate too many rich foods. Now, after two years of hard training, sweat, and discipline I have the build of an 18-year-old and can take pleasure in being mistaken for a college football player. My energy level at work has increased tremendously, and I smile remembering my former belief that bodybuilding would draw away energy needed for my job. There's an improvement in my disposition that has drawn comments from others, and I am more relaxed as a result of getting less involved with petty problems at the office.

My Current Routine

My current routine hasn't changed much. More correctly, it has evolved through fine tuning and adjustments by Franco after discussing my goals, problems, and rate of progress. I continue to run four times a week for a total of eight miles a week and also to walk a minimum of one mile a day. Some weeks I walk a total of 30 miles, and this is done briskly as opposed to a leisurely stroll.

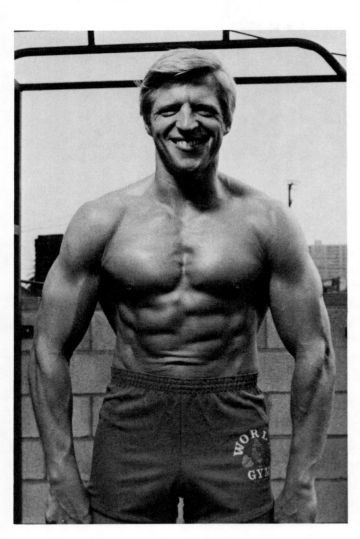

No need to feel embarrassed about not wearing a shirt! Or about compliments from strangers.

Chest Exercises

Incline Dumbbell Bench Press	3 × 10
Incline Barbell Bench Press	3 × 10
Bench Press	3 × 10
Dip	4 × 10
Pullover	3 × 10

Shoulder Exercises

Standing Lateral Raise	7 × 10
Bent-Over Lateral Raise	6 × 10
Standing Barbell Press	3 × 10

Back Exercises

Chin	3 × 8
Pulldown	5 × 10
One-Arm Rowing	2 × 8
Cable Rowing	4 × 8

Arm Exercises

Pressdown	5 × 10
Lying Triceps Bench Press	5 × 10
Lying Triceps Extension	5 × 10
Seated Incline Curl	5 × 10
Preacher Curl	5 × 10
Concentration Curl	1 × 10
Seated Wrist Curl	1 × 25
Standing Wrist Curl	2 × 25

Leg Exercises

Squat	3 × 10
Leg Extension	5 × 25
Leg Curl	2 × 20
Calf Raise	7 × 15

Stomach Exercises

Crunch	4 × 25
Bent-Leg Sit-Up	4 × 25
Side Leg Raise	4 × 25
Side Bend	4 × 25

Training Notes

I begin training by stretching for approximately five minutes to limber up and then start my first chest exercise on the incline bench by using dumbbells to warm the area and gain flexibility. Using light weights for the first set, I gradually increase the poundage, ending the last set with weights quite a bit heavier. Because pressing movements for my shoulders felt uncomfortable in the joints and didn't prove very helpful when I first started out, they were replaced with a higher number of standing lateral raises, begun with 20-pound weights and increased to 35 pounds for the last set. I confess to swinging the weights, but my form is fairly strict since I maintain control of the weight and keep the tension continuous while moving quickly. This procedure is followed by bent-over lateral raises, using 27½-pound dumbbells for the last set of exercises. I have just recently replaced three sets of front raises with standing barbell presses.

Both lateral pulldowns and chins are drawn to the front of my neck rather than the back because the latter movement felt awkward. This change was beneficial because my back has developed extremely well. For one-arm rowing I work with dumbbells as heavy as 70 pounds in addition to using a fantastic cable rowing machine at World Gym. Frequently four sets of leg extensions are all I can manage because the burn is incredible. Franco told me that high repetitions were necessary to achieve the "cuts" that are the foundation for building size. While I know this is true, and will be helpful to others, I believe overly muscular thighs would make me feel uncomfortable in a business suit. Maximum effort is continuously devoted to training my stomach muscles from three to six days a week. Although I ordinarily do 400 repetitions for the abdominal area, sometimes I get through as many as 1,000. My calves grew tremendously this past year of working them hard, giving me a feeling of pride because calf muscles are difficult to build. Throughout my training

sessions I kept thinking of Franco saying, "Train for shape, and size will follow." Just looking at my "before" and "after" pictures proves the soundness of his advice.

Energy Expenditure and Diet

I frequently calculate the number of calories burned up by exercising. For example, I burn off 10 calories a minute by running, which makes a total of 200 calories for going two miles, assuming I run at a relaxed pace of 10-minute miles. Training at the gym, I burn off five calories a minute, or 600 calories after working out two hours. During some exercises I might burn 10–15 calories per minute, but my average of five includes rest periods of 30–60 seconds between sets. Since my ideal weight is maintained with 2,400 calories a day, I can have an additional 600 calories by working out in the gym for two hours. I have learned to eat four or five small meals a day rather than overload myself with food at lunch and dinner. Although I cut down on red meat and fats, my diet contains a fair amount of protein and a good deal of tuna packed in water, white meat, and fish. Since fresh vegetables are fantastic in California, I eat salads often, always careful to limit dressings with oil bases. For a nighttime snack I carve into a pineapple or eat a slice of melon, some grapes, an apple, or an orange.

Actually, I consume a great deal of food, but always with awareness of nutritional values and balancing my diet. After all, I have known the unhappiness of being overweight and out of shape that seems to be an institutionalized problem common in the business world. Unlike many others, I was fortunate in conquering this problem and working my way to physical fitness with my resting pulse rate having dropped from 84 to 60. My blood pressure has gone from 130/90 to 115/78, a remarkable improvement. This does not mean I have completed training but that I have established a new and positive discipline as part of my lifestyle.

A New Goal

A short time ago I was in New York and ran into my old friend, Rock Stonewall, in a health food store. It was quite a reunion because I hadn't seen Rock for 20 years—he's still one of the greatest human beings I've known. When I told him of my experience with Franco Columbu he said it was the smartest thing I could have done. Later on I found a picture of Rock as he looked in 1967 after winning second place for his height class in the Mr. Universe contest. He looked great with a terrific back and shoulders. I told Rock my new goal was becoming as well built as he is. Whenever in New York I train with Rock at the Mid-City Health Club. By following my current pattern of training, Franco has estimated it will take two or three years to reach this new goal.

Time Management Is the Key

I realize that some of my friends in business may think it strange that I am striving to build so much muscle. Certainly, I don't intend to drop out of business and hang out at Muscle Beach all day. Moving up the career ladder is important to me, and I love the excitement of the business world. But Franco has ably managed his multifaceted life of being a doctor of chiropractic and an author as well as appearing in films and television commercials *and* training rigorously. I admire his remarkable management of time, which is the key to being a productive executive.

Despite a busy schedule, weight training and running can be maintained over a lifetime, and, if anything, they seem to slow the aging process. I feel younger in my 30s than I did in my 20s. And Franco, who is in his 40s, has the body of a young athlete in prime condition. This is also true of many other men with demanding schedules, including corporate officers and national leaders who have served as models for me. I plan to continue setting additional short-term workout goals, planning time in my training journal, and taking pictures to check out progress. As I've said before, and repeat again with emphasis, *I'll be working out and maintaining fitness for the remainder of my life.*

I am greatly indebted to Franco for his advice, encouragement, and help in meeting goals I had established. Of course, the hard work of training was mine, as was the discipline of getting up at 5:00 in the morning to leave for the gym when others were sleeping soundly. I had to overcome my nervousness in going to World Gym during those first weeks, comparing my soft and flabby body with others who were firm and muscular. In the beginning I was scared and slowly climbed up the steep stairs leading from World's garage to the gym.

Now I run up the stairs, not worrying, but looking forward to the training session. It has become the only part of the day that is strictly mine with no phones ringing, no kids crying, and no one making demands or asking favors. It's my time, and I love it!

Two

Getting Fit and Staying Fit

Most people are more critical of their own bodies than they are of other men, other women, or the handling of world affairs. This is not surprising since it is fairly easy to get away from other people, and it's only a matter of flipping a switch or dropping a subscription to blot out the news media. There is, however, no getting away from your own body. Even if you go to the moon, where the differing pull of gravity will cause you to weigh less, your body will still be the same shape. And you will still examine it critically, finding the waist too big, the shoulders too narrow, the calves too thin, and so on.

Comprehensive Body Conditioning

This fault finding usually begins in the early teens when you first become aware of your body and begin comparing it with an ideal image, perfectly proportioned and well defined. The fact is that no one has a perfect body, but many have created this illusion by doing exercises that bring the entire body into balance. While most sports exercise *certain* muscles, only bodybuilding affords the comprehensive conditioning needed to tailor your body for the precise results you want.

For example, if your only exercise is bicycling or running, you will lose fat, trim your waist, and develop good thighs and calves. However, the upper part of your body will remain essentially the same. If your arms are thin or your shoulders narrow, they will then be out of

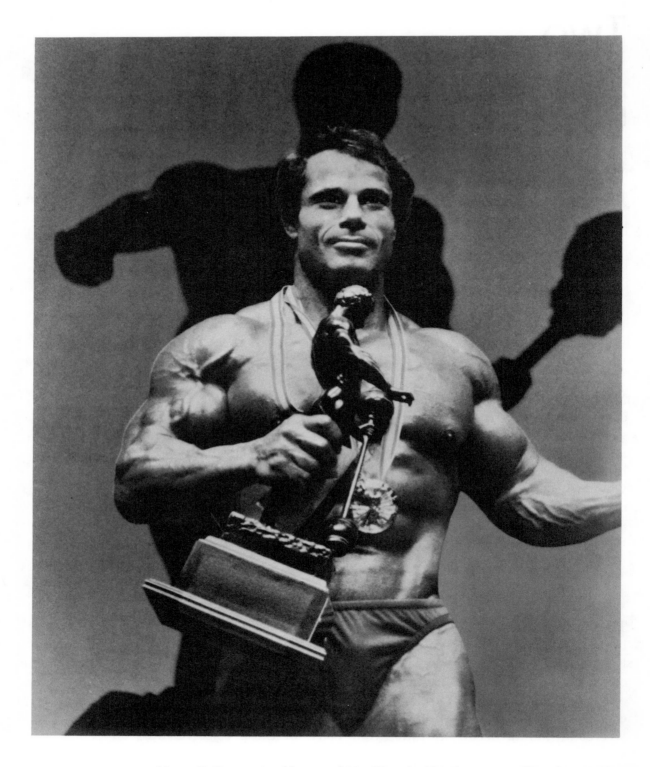

At age 40, Franco won his second Mr. Olympia title. Five years earlier, after winning his first Olympia title, he injured his left knee so severely many friends thought he could never compete again. His knowledge of kinesiology and his patience helped him slowly recover until he was once again in competitive shape.

proportion with the well-developed and finely conditioned lower half of your body. The same problem is true of most other sports since they require you to play in a standing position.

On the other hand, bodybuilding, and working with weight resistance equipment, has you squatting, sitting, lying on an incline, and lying prone. Not only does your entire body undergo comprehensive muscle conditioning, but your blood supply is dispersed to every part of your body during a single workout. This is another advantage over sports such as tennis, soccer, and running, during which the blood supply goes mainly to the legs. The important difference in blood circulation during weight training exercises is perhaps best exemplified by doing a bench press, when a tremendous influx of blood goes to the chest and shoulders and from there to the neck and on to the brain. In this way, the brain receives the supply of oxygen needed to function at high capacity either on the job or away from it.

Muscle-Building Myths

Beginning a new lifestyle, in this case the health and fitness lifestyle, is always difficult. People tend to look for excuses not to change and if enough people spread these excuses around, the excuse often becomes a "fact." In reality, such a "fact" is just a myth that supports the status quo. I would like to explore several myths concerning the development of muscles and getting into shape.

Bodybuilding Makes Men Muscle-Bound

Many men say, "I don't want too many muscles" or "I don't want to become muscle-bound." Some believe that several months of weight-lifting will certainly turn them into Tarzan. If this were actually possible they would make a fortune selling their secret to bodybuilders around the world.

It is extremely difficult to develop the muscularity of a bodybuilding champion. To get my muscles into contest shape I must train for two or three hours a day at top level for two or three months. Out of 25 million who train with weights in the United States, only about 2,000 enter competitions. Of this number only a few achieve the muscularity necessary to become champions. One or two receive a great deal of publicity, yet, on seeing these unique individuals, many men assume they will develop the same muscularity within a month or two of lifting their first dumbbell. They never stop to consider that only one or two men out of 25 million have achieved championship status after many years of discipline and training.

All That Muscle Will Turn into Fat

Another popularly believed myth is that any muscle gained will turn into fat when bodybuilding workouts are stopped or cut down. *This is impossible, because fat and muscle are completely different substances.* Fat and muscle are composed of different types of cells that exist in the body in isolation from each other. Fat is a semisolid organic compound. Muscle is made up of bundles of fibers, totally incompatible for conversion into fat.

Muscularity is acquired only by training and by eating protein foods such as fish, eggs, and meat. Fat is gained by not training or exercising and by eating fattening foods such as bacon and sausage, which contain a high percentage of animal fat, and all foods containing sugar.

Many former athletes become fat because they formed eating habits based on the huge caloric requirements of their active days. For instance, football players train hard for two or three hours a day, eating enormous amounts of food because their goal is to become big and muscular. After leaving the sport competitively, however, they lose sight of the fact that their intake of food should be decreased. For this reason many football players become fat when they retire from the game.

The myth that bodybuilding will make you muscle-bound is also based on the confusion between fat and muscle. Athletes who become "muscle-bound"—that is, those who have lost freedom of movement in some body parts—more accurately are fat-bound. It is actually the accumulation of fat between muscles that causes the problem. Approximately 40–50 percent of surplus weight is made up of fat, accumulating between the muscles and interfering with their freedom of action. By working hard on building muscles you will avoid becoming muscle-bound and achieve more strength and flexibility.

During my years as a boxer I trained regularly with weights and became the lightweight boxing champion of Italy. It is well known that boxing requires fighters to be fast and loose. If weight training had slowed me down, or interfered with my freedom of action, winning the championship would have been impossible. This experience exemplifies the fact that weight training is a good basis for achieving the endurance and muscular strength needed for any sport.

Only Young Men Can Start Bodybuilding

Another concern most often expressed in mail received from this country and around the world is that some men consider themselves too old to start bodybuilding. I am always happy to inform them that bodybuilding is one sport that recognizes no age barriers. It is possible to start training without weights at the age of six or seven and continue until the age of 100. It is even possible to start working out at the age of 95, though anyone over age 40 would be wise to consult a physician before undertaking any new form of strenuous exercise.

At my chiropractic clinic there are four or five old men who are on a training program. One of these delightful men is 96, and he trains for two hours every morning, doing free-weight exercises together with others using very light weights. He earnestly devotes his time to this daily workout because he enjoys it above all else. Several others are also into their later years. One is 75, another is 78, and others are over 65. All began to develop muscles in their old age. Being highly pleased by their progress, they walk into my office most anxious to take off their shirts and show me their muscles. "Just look at my biceps!" they proudly shout.

Muscular potential will develop according to your age, with the maximum capacity for growth occurring between the ages of 15 and 40. During these years you can develop 100 percent of your muscular potential. After the age of 40 this percentage begins decreasing slowly as follows.

Development of Potential	Age
90%	40–50
65–90%	50–60
40–70%	60–70
20–40%	70–80

After the age of 80 you can continue developing 20 percent of your muscles for the remainder of your life.

As you get older it is important to use more corrective exercises designed to improve the posture of the body and to balance muscles for equal strength. It is also necessary to use lighter weights because it takes longer to warm up. Muscles need to be stretched due to a certain amount of rigidity. Running and bicycling should be done at an easy pace, but you can train for longer periods than in your youth. In older years the focus is not on building muscles but on achieving a good muscle balance at a steady rate. While training there should be no feeling of discomfort in your joints or other areas of your body, so each session becomes an event you look forward to with pleasure.

The Benefits of Shaping Up

If you didn't think there were benefits to shaping up, I'm sure you wouldn't have bought this book. Nevertheless, I would like to discuss them to ensure you have a complete understanding. Hopefully, with such an understanding, your desire to shape up will grow. This desire begins the snowball effect of getting you into an exercise program; once in, you will begin to *feel* the benefits of shaping up. Once you've got the feeling, you won't quit because you'll like the feeling and desire to feel that way all the time.

Strength and Stamina

All my training programs increase stamina and strength. Stamina is measured by the speed of a movement and the number of times it can be performed without stopping. The key to increasing stamina is to train hard and fast, forcing your body to do more than usual until it adapts to the added strain and can handle it.

Strength results from the exertion of a single force against an object and is measured by the amount of time an activity can be sustained by a particular set of muscles. By increasing the amount of weight lifted every week or month you will make your muscles work harder. As they adapt to the added resistance your muscles will grow and become stronger. Therefore, when the notation 1×20 or 2×10 is given for the number of times an exercise is performed, this means you will continue doing the same number of sets and reps but with heavier weights to develop your muscular strength.

In the beginning your body may rebel when it is forced to work harder. Muscles weakened by years of sedentary living will revolt against the additional exertion. You may find it necessary to fight impulses commanding you to put the weights down and rest or to do the exercises out of the given order with the easier ones at the end of the training session. You may find any number of reasons to skip an entire training session if you don't stop to remember how good you felt after the last one.

Those who are strong enjoy living in their bodies because the pleasure of physical power is always with them and under their control. It is not dependent on the economy, the weather, or the whims of others. In all probability the time invested in developing strength and stamina will add years to your life. Most certainly it will provide the immediate gratification of adding hours to your day. Too often people feel cheated out of life when they do nothing more exciting after a day's work than flop down on the couch and watch television. They look forward only to weekends or annual vacations to live fully. But if you can develop your strength and stamina, another five or six hours of productive living can be given over to sports, dancing, or classes. Many have devoted these extra hours to turning a hobby into a livelihood, becoming their own boss and doing work they love.

By considering the roles that strength and stamina play in your life you will come to realize that almost every act is made simpler by a strong body. In the morning you will get up with energy left over from the previous day. Knowing that you are unusually strong will give you a feeling of confidence as you tackle the multitude of problems that can crop up in the course of a day's work.

Strength and stamina are qualities to be desired and developed by everyone, not just athletes and marines ready for combat duty. A more durable body forms the foundation for a happier, better adjusted life, putting you on the road to discovering your level of peak performance.

Weight Gain

If you are too thin and want to gain weight, it is important to gear yourself toward gaining muscle rather than fat. The important difference between the two is illustrated clearly by some bodybuilders and powerlifters who are so big and bulked up that their manner of walking leads people to believe they are muscle-bound. This impression is not due to their muscle mass but to the accumulation of a great deal of fat on their bodies.

The key to overcoming thinness lies in putting on muscle weight rather than fat and exercising with weights as heavy as possible to build up an acceptable amount of musculature. Ten pounds of muscle gained yearly is the maximum amount to set for a goal. Ideally, gaining no more than five or six pounds will ensure that your weight gain is pure muscle.

The most important foods for gaining muscle weight are eggs and fish because they are low in fat and high in protein, not necessarily the protein powders that many people use. I recommend raising your caloric intake but to avoid stuffing yourself with foods of no nutritional value. Care should be taken to maintain a balanced diet with a variety of foods (meat, fish, vegetables, fruits, etc.) to obtain the necessary amount of each of the six basic nutrients. Since the main function of carbohydrates is to supply energy to the body, you should eat carbohydrate sources before going to the gym. The carbs found in fresh fruit, for example, provide just what your body needs before a workout.

Do not overload your system by eating three large meals a day. It is far better to have smaller portions of food five times daily. The trick behind gaining muscle weight lies in eating every three or four hours. When more time elapses between meals the protein in the stomach is digested, causing the body to draw protein energy from the muscles. This will cause them to decrease in size. Therefore, be attentive to keeping a certain measure of protein in the body so your muscles are fed at all times.

Weight Reduction

When it comes to weight reduction the basic principles of training regularly and monitoring food intake still apply but in a different way. As previously mentioned, those who want to lose weight will exercise using light weights and do a high number of sets and reps to burn off fat deposits. The number of calories they consume will depend greatly on the amount of time and energy devoted to training sessions.

Some men are concerned about working out regularly because they are afraid of becoming too muscular. For some reason they picture themselves developing the physique of championship bodybuilders after a short time of training with barbells and dumbbells, as if this equipment were imbued with the same magical qualities that made Jack's beanstalk grow sky-high overnight. Yet the same men would not believe themselves capable of achieving the champion status of a golfer or baseball player without devoting many years of their lives to training hard and perfecting their technique. Bodybuilding means exactly what it says: you build muscles over a period of time, shaping and contouring your body for the precise look you want. At all times the results are completely under your control since muscle potential is developed only by training with very heavy weights. If you work with light weights, your muscles will increase slightly in size as you improve their tone and gain stamina, strength, and energy. So don't worry about getting too muscular; instead devote your energy to losing fat.

The Solution to Crash Dieting

There are several methods of losing weight when you combine regular training with an awareness of food intake. Bear in mind that one hour of very hard training will burn off approximately 1,000 calories. If you are not consuming 2,500 calories daily and gaining weight, you can still maintain this diet provided you work out for one hour and burn off 1,000 calories. You will stop gaining and slowly lose weight. For faster results, reduce your food intake to 2,000 calories and thereby increase your rate of weight loss without going on a severe diet.

Too often people go on crash diets because they promise a rapid weight loss without the need for exercise. When this type of plan is followed you lose both muscle and fat, leaving your skin loose and lacking muscle tone. Although the weight loss will make you look smaller, you will retain the fat because weak and flabby muscles cannot break up fat deposits and move them out of your system. When fat settles around muscles they stretch and sag, causing surrounding tissue to sag. The only way to bring these muscles back into shape is to exercise.

Allergic Reactions

The solution to reducing weight and maintaining the loss does not lie in strict diets but in your awareness of what particular foods do to your body. In general, the most important foods are easily digested; they will be discussed further in Chapter 5.

Another factor contributing to weight loss is the elimination of foods that are allergens. Perhaps you eat a great deal of chicken because it is high in protein and not very fattening. However, an allergy to chicken can cause you to gain weight when eating it. By listening to your body it is possible to gain insights regarding foods that cause allergic reactions. Perhaps your breathing changes and becomes heavy or your sinus passages clog after you eat dairy products, beer, or processed foods. Another symptom is feeling bloated for too long a time after eating and then immediately becoming hungry again. By eliminating fattening foods and those causing allergic reactions you will lose weight very quickly.

Above all, remember that the body is not a machine programmed to lose weight according to a rigorous schedule. Your weight loss will even out in the long run, but the body will take its own time. Do not weigh yourself every day, expecting to see a uniform amount of weight loss. It is far better to weigh yourself once a week or every 10 days. After all, it has taken you years or perhaps decades to become overweight, so you can't expect your body to reach a new equilibrium overnight.

The Weight-Loss Menu presented on page 30 is a diet that will help you lose weight quickly without causing any nutritional deficiencies. It was developed to complement any weight training program you choose. To judge the number of calories you can burn off with a particular routine, figure on losing approximately 1,000 calories with the more advanced programs and from 600 to 900 calories with the others, depending on how hard you train and the rest periods allowed between sets.

Weight-Loss Menu

Breakfast

- 2 eggs, cooked any style
- a small dish of fresh pineapple *or* half a papaya *or* ¼ pound of grapes
- 1 cup of coffee

The fruit should be eaten after and not before the eggs for proper digestion. Juice is not necessary because you are having fresh fruit.

Lunch

- fish, either grilled or broiled
- a plate of salad
- 1 or 2 glasses of wine *or* 1 glass of beer

Use no mayonnaise or butter on the fish. You can add salt and pepper; however, salt isn't necessary since fish contains its own salt. The salad should not be eaten before the fish but along with it or immediately afterward— again, for proper digestion.

Dinner

- fish, either grilled or broiled, *or* chicken, either grilled or broiled, with the skin removed
- a plate of salad
- 1 glass of wine

Your usual vitamins or minerals can be taken before, during, or after meals. It is important to increase your mineral intake since you will not eat a great variety of food. If the mineral content of the body drops below a certain level, this can cause the problems that make so many diets dangerous.

Training regularly and following this diet will make your weight loss rapid.

Training Equipment and Facilities

It is a common belief that jogging, bicycling, and tennis are inexpensive sports, but in the long run they are more expensive than bodybuilding. When you buy weights they last forever, unlike jogging shoes, which must be purchased every few months at the cost of $40–$100 per pair. Playing tennis also requires expensive shoes, good rackets, restringing costs, and court fees. And it's hardly likely that someone will steal your barbell or dumbbells as readily or easily as an expensive bicycle.

Despite stormy weather, which stops you from playing tennis or bicycling, you can easily train at home or in the office because only a small amount of space is needed to work out. In the privacy of your own home there's rarely any competition, so you can discover your own potential rather than waste time comparing your progress with that of others.

Weights are not required for exercising the stomach, hips, or thighs. A sit-up board is not necessary for abdominal exercises. As a matter of fact, they quite often contribute to lower back problems. In the first program I demonstrate stomach exercises that I used to get into shape for the Mr. Olympia contest. These were done without the dubious benefit of a sit-up board.

At the start, a minor investment of $10–$20 will provide you with one pair of 10-pound dumbbells that can be used for doing more than 50 exercises for different parts of the body.

Clothing is also simple and inexpensive. In general, either it should be loose fitting or it should stretch with body movements. When the weather is cold, be sure to wear a warm-up suit to prevent your body from getting hot while exercising and then cold as you walk around. Take additional time to warm up so you feel loose and start with movements geared to improve circulation and therefore avoid injury. The key to progressing quickly through the day's set of exercises, whether in summer or winter, lies in keeping the muscles warm.

If you live in a cold climate, where the temperature changes drastically from overheated living areas to frigid basements and garages, I recommend training only when wearing a warm-up suit. During warm weather you can work out dressed in a tank top or T-shirt and shorts.

No specific weight is required for training shoes. Those used for running are fine unless you begin lifting heavy weights. Then very strong shoes are needed to provide a firm base of support.

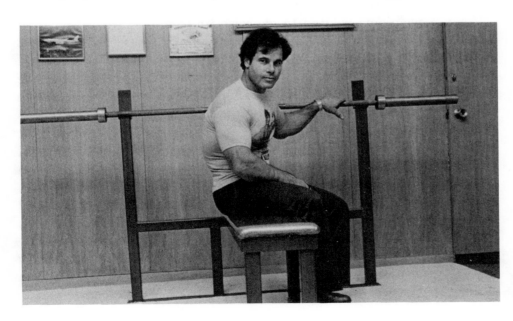

This barbell is capable of holding hundreds of pounds.

The equipment you purchase will vary according to your budget and seriousness of intention. Later in this chapter are several lists of equipment geared to accommodate different needs and goals, ranging from a few pieces of basic equipment to a complete home gym ranging in cost from $1,000 to $5,000. I suggest beginning simply and adding equipment as you progress.

The Exercise Machine

Some beginners, unfamiliar with the advantages of working with free weights, become captivated by the idea of buying one of the exercise machines advertised in newspapers and magazines. The sleek architecture of the unit inspires them with a feeling of efficiency and getting things done right. Promises made by the manufacturer seem to offer the ultimate solution for keeping in shape without wasting time.

The price of $500 or more for an exercise unit guaranteed to last five years appears to be a good investment, particularly when compared to the cost of a one-year membership at a health spa or gym. Some may even consider the machine a greater bargain, believing the entire family will profit by having the unit at home.

While many of the better models are good, none is good enough for a home gym unless supplemented by free weight equipment. Through the years I have tried all the exercise machines myself, even the most sophisticated models now being used by professional football teams. This experience convinced me that none can match the benefits gained from using free weights.

Certain problems related to exercise units will not be discovered until a unit is purchased. They will surface only when the machine is at home and you have been using it for several months. For instance, after two or three months of doing the same 10–20 exercises on the same machine you will find that doing all your exercises on one machine is boring. If you sometimes feel like a robot on the job, it is likely you will experience a similar feeling using the exercise unit. At that point you might move it out to the garage, promising yourself to use it again when the time is right. However, the machine soon will start rusting under an accumulation of old tires, rotting garden hoses, broken screens, and other junk usually stored in garages. And you won't be in good shape either, letting your complete home gym rust away as you continue paying the monthly installment charges.

Another disadvantage in using only the machine is that after several months of great improvement all progress will come to a standstill. When muscles and muscle groups become accustomed to the same exercise, no further progress can be made. Your muscles, like your mind, need the stimulation that comes from a new source such as a different exercise or a new program.

If you continue exercising regularly, you will maintain your earlier success but will be unable to advance. This can be disheartening, since man is a rational creature who needs to see positive results from dedication and hard work. Discouraged, he may give up the entire notion of exercise and devote his free time and attention to electronic games. However, free weights give you a choice among exercises for each body part, allowing muscle growth and development to continue.

A final consideration is that machines can cause injuries unless you know precisely what you are doing. For the past 10 years I've worked with thousands of athletes at my clinic and found that most of their injuries were caused by exercise machines. Unlike dumbbells, which allow the joints a free range of motion, the machine is a fixed piece of equipment unable to accommodate your unique body structure. Because they restrict movement, forcing joints to bend according to the machines' limitations, friction is caused and injuries can occur.

Even if a perfect exercise unit were built for a particular body, it would not be entirely suitable for another. Human beings are not yet cloned like photocopies of office memos. Certainly, they are not constructed like cars on assembly lines, with all parts of one model interchangeable with those of another. There are more than 4 billion people in the world, and like fingerprints, no two bodies are structured alike. Research has shown that even twins are not the same.

Starting a Home Gym

Two pairs of dumbbells, priced about $20 each, are sufficient for starting a gym at home. I recommend getting one set that weighs 10 pounds and another weighing 20. In the beginning some body parts will be weak, so you will be unable to lift the heavier weights. Others will be strong and would gain little benefit from the lighter pair. Buy fixed dumbbells rather than those with adjustable weights and clamps because the clamps eventually fail, making it necessary to buy another set. Also, muscles and muscle groups tend to cool down in the time spent adjusting clamps. The blood pumped into muscles will partially drain off, defeating the purpose of your workout.

As your training advances, purchase a barbell with about 50 pounds of weight. Priced at $50–$70, they come in several sizes. I suggest getting a short bar; five feet is as good a size for training as the longer bars and is easier to manipulate in the home.

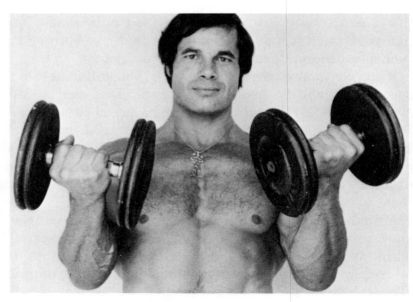

Fixed-weight dumbbells are the best investment over the long run.

If you want to expand your gym with additional equipment, buy a bench, chinning bar, squat rack, and a preacher curl bench. These pieces cost an average of about $100 each. Bear in mind that the equipment will last a lifetime and is a solid investment. Most of these pieces are usually available at J.C. Penney and Sears stores.

Home Gym for $500

This type of gym is totally suitable for the more advanced programs, beginning with program 4.

- 3 sets of dumbbells weighing 10, 20, and 30 pounds each
- 1 barbell, 5 or 6 feet long
- 4 sets of plates (weights) for the barbell, weighing 2½, 5, 10, and 20 pounds each
- 1 bench, adjustable for regular bench press exercises and those requiring an incline bench

Additional pieces of equipment can be purchased according to your budget and measure of progress. For those who want to build and strengthen thigh muscles, I recommend a leg extension machine priced between $300 and $400. If your spending money or room for working out is limited, you may prefer to buy an attachment for the bench that makes it adaptable for leg extensions and leg curls.

A chinning bar is important for stretching the spine and doing advanced back exercises. The type that attaches to the ceiling is ideal and will cost from $15 to $30. Also, one can be built in the backyard

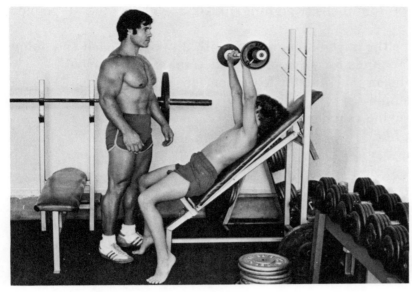

A weight bench as shown can be used for a variety of exercises in a variety of positions.

with plumbing supplies. A bar that fits into a doorway is better than nothing, but one allowing a wide grip will produce optimum results, particularly for stretching back muscles.

For an additional $50 you can have the convenience of a squat rack, a highly useful piece of equipment for removing weight from your back after finishing the squatting exercises. And when you can afford it, buy another barbell and extra weights. In this way the bar with lighter weights can be used on the bench press and the heavier barbell on the squat rack. Time spent changing weights not only cools off your muscles, as mentioned, but also interrupts the rhythm of your training routine.

The Complete Home Gym

The complete gym described here costs more than $1,000, with some additional pieces ranging in price from $1,000 to $5,000. This includes all the equipment you could possibly need, even if you later intend to get into heavy training:

- bench for regular bench exercises and bench presses
- incline bench for incline bench presses
- squat rack
- preacher bench for curls
- cable machine for all types of pulls
- 2 barbells, at least 6–7 feet long
- 1 barbell, 5 feet long
- 1 triceps bar, actually a curling bar used for triceps exercises

- 6 pairs of dumbbells, weighing 10, 20, 25, 30, 35, and 40 pounds each·
- plates for the barbell, beginning with 2½ pounds each and going up to 45 pounds for an approximate total of 500 pounds
- leg extension machine for leg extensions and leg curls
- calf machine
- T-bar rowing machine
- dipping bar
- chinning bar
- stationary bicycle

If you can spend an additional $3,000–$6,000, a Universal Gym machine is highly recommended for all types of exercises. As mentioned earlier, however, the machine does not eliminate the need for free-weight equipment because it does not allow you to vary exercises.

With all this equipment you can work out in two ways: (1) train your entire body during each session as described in Program 6 (see page 87), or (2) train four days a week, exercising half of the body on one day and the other half at the next session, as explained in Program 7 (see page 88).

How to Choose and Use a Gym

In the United States there are more than 10 different types of gymnasiums, ranging from those found in high schools to totally machine-furnished gyms using Nautilus, Universal, or Paramount equipment. These various types and the facilities they offer fall into the following five categories.

High School Gyms

High school gyms involved in community service programs are open to the public in the evening and sometimes during the summer. They are usually equipped with barbells and dumbbells and perhaps a few benches. Some may have a Universal Gym machine.

YMCA and Other Community-Oriented Clubs

Prepared to serve the community at large, these clubs have gyms with every kind of free-weight equipment, in addition to facilities for other sports, including swimming, basketball, boxing, and track.

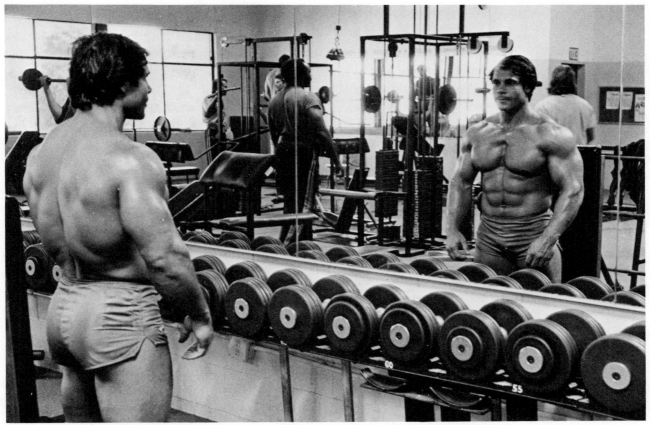

Commercial gyms provide the state of the art in equipment, mirrors by which you can check for strict exercise form, and the advice and encouragement of others.

Instructors teach classes in gymnastics, aerobics, yoga, and other physical education activities.

Health Spas

Usually the equipment at a spa is mixed, with free weights and machines manufactured by different companies. Most men working out at spas use both types. The facilities vary, but most have exercise classes, saunas, and steam rooms; more expensive clubs usually have swimming pools, racquetball courts, and sometimes indoor running tracks.

Machine-Equipped Gyms

Although a few may have barbells and dumbbells, the majority of these have only machines such as the Nautilus models. You train by moving from one machine to another.

Professional Bodybuilding Gymnasiums

Here you will find the ultimate in powerlifting equipment. Most is free-weight equipment, the type competitive bodybuilders like to use. In addition, you will find a number of heavy-duty machines hand-constructed by the owners. Professional and noncompetitive bodybuilders train here, as do men concerned with serious exercise either for health reasons or to condition their bodies for other sports. The staff is highly experienced in hard training that brings quick results.

Checking Out Gyms

Before joining a gym, check out several facilities in your area, comparing fees, equipment, and other furnishings that may be important to you. Take into consideration the distance you must travel, remembering that you will work out three days a week, or perhaps four if you decide on a split routine. A gym located a half hour from home may seem to offer more, but one that is closer could prove far easier to attend regularly.

Since atmosphere can be highly conducive to—or incompatible with—maintaining enthusiasm and training regularly, it, too, should be considered. The professional bodybuilding gymnasium, being strictly utilitarian, is packed with heavy weights. Rarely is anything chrome-plated. The equipment found here is the best available since it is well balanced and maintained. Because many of those training are competing professionals, their advice far surpasses any given in a health spa.

In contrast, gyms geared for a more social environment have thick carpeting, chrome-plated machines, coffee shops, and sun decks. You may be more comfortable in these surroundings, particularly if you are gregarious and you enjoy socializing after training. Although the equipment is usually inferior to that found in professional bodybuilding gymnasiums, the workouts are approximately the same unless you intend to become a competitive bodybuilder.

Some men who are machine devotees may prefer to work out with Nautilus equipment exclusively. The advantage of machine-equipped gyms is having many athletes train simultaneously, and the safety factor is another plus. For example, you can pick up bench-press apparatus and, if it feels uncomfortable, let it go without harming yourself.

I recommend any health club or gymnasium that has both machines and free-weight equipment, since the combination of both affords the greatest freedom of choice. As you become experienced, gaining strength and developing muscular potential, you can progress to advanced programs without concern for the availability of equipment needed to reach new goals.

Cost. Prices will vary according to the competition among clubs and gyms and special deals offered for five-year memberships. Because some gyms tend to fold shortly after giving half-price deals, be certain to choose one that will be in operation the full term of membership. Usually, state- and city-funded gyms are far less expensive than privately owned gyms. For example the Venice Beach Gym has equipment that is moved outside during the day and returned indoors at night. The fee for joining this state-supported club is only $20 a year. In comparison, commercial gyms range in price from $150 to more than $1,000 yearly, with some exclusive health clubs charging $1,000 for membership plus additional fees for using certain facilities.

Availability of Equipment. To avoid the disappointment and frustration of joining a gym or health spa and later discovering that its equipment is not suited to your needs, review the training programs that follow and decide which are best for you. Since some of my routines are intended specifically for gym use, take this book along when you are checking them out. Don't hesitate to show instructors the programs and ask if their gym is equipped for the one you have chosen. Beware of slick operators calling themselves physical fitness consultants who will promise anything to get you to sign a contract. For this reason it is important to acquire as much knowledge as possible about the right training program for your body. To know as much as possible is power and strength in itself.

Because free-weight exercises work on the principle of weight resistance, many adapt to machine equipment. A lateral raise, for example, can be done either with dumbbells or by using a Nautilus machine. The only difference is the angle of movement. Pulldowns can also be done on several types of machines, provided they work the same muscle. If a movement feels uncomfortable while you are using any apparatus, be alert to the fact that you can be injured by friction caused in the joints. When the movement does not feel strained or awkward, but free and flowing, you know a specific machine is right for you.

Trial Workouts. Because hands-on experience is invaluable, ask for a trial workout at several gyms to acquire a working knowledge of their equipment and facilities. Usually they are happy to accommodate you and allow one free of charge, but at some you may be asked to pay a slight fee. Afterward, when you are at home and away from the pitch of a high-powered "fitness consultant," you can make up your mind.

Concentration. A problem encountered in a spa or gym is that sometimes there is too much socializing and not enough hard training. Not only do you run the danger of being injured by lack of concentration, but rapid progress requires you to focus on the particular body part being exercised. When it comes to weight training, or any other sport, concentration and improvement are synonymous.

To test this point, a parallel study was run between two men of similar build and approximate weight. They trained with identical weights, doing the same number of sets and reps. One man was permitted to let his attention wander while the other concentrated on his muscles, movement, and form. Although both men went through the same motions, only the man who concentrated showed improvement because his energy was not directed away from the parts of his body being exercised. Keep in mind that a direct link is formed between the muscles worked and your brain during any specific exercise.

Advantages. Once you have considered the options presented and joined a gym or health spa, the benefits gained are well worth the cost of membership if you attend regularly. The advantage of having an assortment of equipment from which to choose and all different weights of dumbbells and barbells at hand will encourage you to try programs that are increasingly difficult. Also, the energy generated by those working out in a gym can be stimulating on days when your vitality is low and you don't feel like working out. Just walking through the door and seeing everyone exercising can effectively draw you away from any problems that have drained your own energy. There are numerous other advantages, including the opportunity to learn from those who are more advanced and finding others to share your interest in getting fit. Some friendships formed in gyms or health clubs last a lifetime.

Exercising at the Gym

The best time to join a gym is after you have done some training at home. If this proves impossible, you can still learn enough to use a gym without wasting time by reading several books on bodybuilding to familiarize yourself with the equipment, the terminology of weight training, and a variety of programs.

As previously mentioned, gym instructors are usually present to guide you through the early sessions, particularly the first. Some may devote a half hour or more to explaining the equipment and correcting your form as you move through the exercises. Within a week, however, new members will make claims on the instructor's time, leaving him no time to concern himself with your form or problems with equipment. To have one question answered may require trotting around after the instructor for 10–15 minutes until he finishes conducting a newcomer through his paces. Being left to fend for yourself with nothing but a program card listing the exercises can be disconcerting, especially for beginners. You may be wondering if dumbbells should be held with an overgrip or undergrip when exercising the biceps or exactly how to position your hands for a reverse grip on a barbell.

To assure a successful workout at each session I strongly urge you to take this book to the gym and use it as a reference guide. The correct form for each exercise is shown throughout the book and in the glossary, together with precise explanations defining each movement from start to finish. Close-ups are provided to show the proper grip and positioning of the hands when lifting weights because this is necessary for making progress and preventing injuries. Weak or incorrect grips hamper an increase in muscle strength and can force the body out of alignment during exercises.

In every program I took into account the necessity to balance exercises among all muscles so they will become equally strong and well developed. Many important factors such as these are beyond the scope of most gym instructors since they lack my background as a professional bodybuilder and doctor of chiropractic. Therefore, this book will serve as a valuable tool at the gym if you also take along a good supply of concentration, discipline, determination, and patience.

Special Training Considerations

Many of those in training move steadily toward their goals and then hit a plateau, where progress comes to a halt. The enthusiasm they once felt dies down. Some, not seeing any results from all their dedication, sweat, and hard work, may believe they have reached their limitations. At this point it is vital to remember that the power in you is limited only by your belief in its limitation.

Plateaus

Every goal-oriented person, whether in sports, business, politics, or the arts, has suffered the experience of being stranded on a plateau. During my years of training I have faced this problem more than once and have overcome it each time, using one method or another and sometimes a combination of several. Realizing this problem was not uniquely mine, I included in this book a variety of programs to lift you from those plateaus and put you back on the road to reaching your goals. The following suggestions are drawn from my years of experience. They have made me a winner many times over and brought me to the ultimate goal of world champion.

- Change programs every two to four months.
- Change the time of day you work out.
- Speed up the exercise pace, moving faster and more aggressively with shorter rest periods between sets.
- Use another program.
- Keep the same program, but exchange exercises for others that work the same muscle or muscle groups.

In addition, I have found that going to another gym can prove greatly valuable. When training for the Mr. Olympia contest, I worked out in four gyms and also at home. In this way my body was constantly exposed to new and different movements that stimulated and energized my muscles.

Breakthroughs

When you achieve greater results than expected from your training, the program you are following is the right one for your body. Continue using this program for as long as possible, but occasionally switch to another program to make different demands on your body for a month or two. Both the mind and muscles need a break from routine and are stimulated by a new challenge.

On the Road

Travel should not greatly interfere with your workout program since most exercises needed to stay fit can easily be done in your hotel room. For instance, push-ups, which are still among the best exercises for strengthening the muscles of the chest, shoulders, and triceps (back of the arm) can be done by utilizing two chairs found in any hotel room. Hamstring stretches also can be done by using one of the chairs, and all stomach and hip exercises are done on the floor even in the gym.

Two pieces of lightweight equipment can be packed in a suitcase and taken along with you. One is a jump rope for working the leg muscles, and the other, used for exercising the upper body, is a long piece of expandable rubber that folds into a small rectangle so it can be carried even in an attaché case. The accompanying photo shows exercises using this tool.

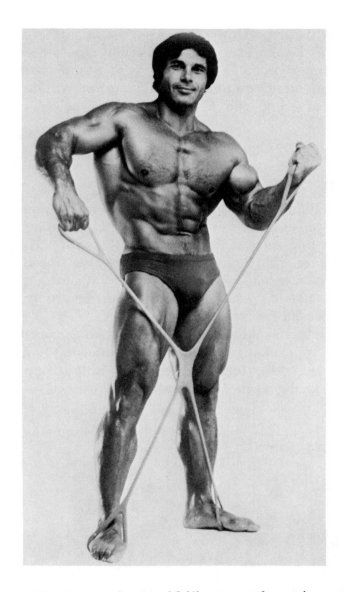

This exercise device is portable and increases the stress of stretching exercises.

For those who would like to work out in a gym while on a business trip, a number of major hotels now have in-house health clubs complete with gym equipment, saunas, steam room, and jacuzzis. To find out which hotels provide these facilities, call your travel agent or ask someone in the travel department of your organization to make the arrangements.

If your job takes you off the beaten track and you feel like training in a gym, one can be found in any town of moderate size by looking in the yellow pages of the phone book. In most cases you can drive right over without calling ahead. When you go in, simply say you are in town for only a couple of days and would like to work out. Usually you will be allowed to train free of charge or for a minimal fee of about $5 for one session.

You will be enriched by the experience of working out in a different environment in any of the thousands of gyms found across the United States and in foreign countries. Working with dumbbells, barbells, bench presses, and other equipment familiar to you will do much to make you feel at home and dispel feelings of being a stranger alone on the road.

Training with a Partner

For those who find it difficult to achieve the discipline of regular workouts or to complete an exercise routine, I suggest a training partner. Perhaps you can find several friends to join the gym with you. Keep in mind, however, that training with more than three others will make your workouts too slow. Be careful not to choose a training partner who has a sour view of life because his negativity will drain you of energy needed for training.

Ideally, you and your partner should be equally motivated to shape up and friendly enough to exchange constructive criticism. For example, you can watch each other for progress in smoothly lifting and lowering weight by facing each other and using two sets of

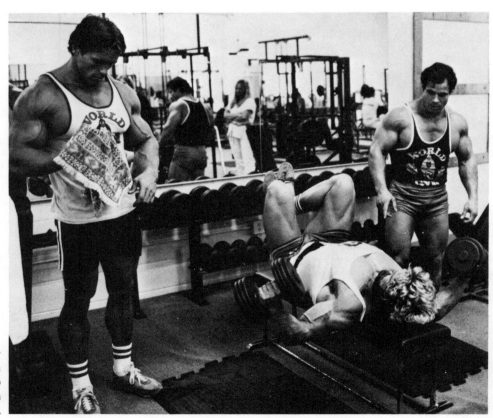

Arnold Schwarzenegger and Franco watch European superstar Jusup Wilkosz perform Dumbbell Bench presses.

dumbbells. Another benefit is having a friend ready to spot you when doing bench presses and squats. Or your partner can use the Exercise Glossary at the back of this book to make certain that you are using the proper form and grip to prevent injuries.

I found that working out with the right partner helped me reach all my bodybuilding goals. Arnold Schwarzenegger and I have trained together since we met in Europe. Yes, we had fun and made a game of training, but we never forgot to push each other to our maximums. He made me do extra sets when I didn't feel like it; I pushed him into lifting heavy weights by going into them myself and forcing him to follow suit. This is what I mean about finding the right partner.

The bad news about training with someone is becoming so dependent on your partner that you are tempted to skip your own workout if he doesn't show up at the gym. He is also likely to take vacations, to go off on business trips, or even to be transferred to another state, leaving you floundering without his support. Therefore, it is vital always to have your own goals in mind, keeping a training diary similar to Rick Newcombe's (see Chapter 1) to provide the stimulus you need to keep you on course.

Training Tips

Throughout this book are many tips on training I discovered over the years, which will assure you of getting maximal results in a short time. We all know that there are a number of ways to train, but too often men become discouraged when they observe little progress. Every day I receive letters from several individuals telling me of their lack of success with training programs before following my routines and suggestions. I learned how to get into shape the hard way, so I can pass on a lot of experiences.

1. Always use the first 10 minutes of your workout to warm up. Many people train incorrectly, training their stomach and hips before doing their weight training exercises, for example. Working the abdominals at the outset of a session is a waste of time because the body and stomach muscles are still cold. It is not surprising that so many men become discouraged or, even worse, injure themselves.

As you work out your temperature will rise and you will begin sweating. Within an hour your body will be properly warmed up, and you will get quick results from the abdominal exercises done at the end of each session. This method will also help prevent back problems.

2. Each muscle group requires from one to five exercises. The more exercises per body part, the better trained that part becomes. On the average it is desirable to use two exercises for each part so training is more intensive. Bodybuilders who are in training for competition use four to five exercises per body part.

3. Every body has strong and weak points. Some people have strong, well-developed legs but skinny arms. These individuals should do one exercise for the legs and thighs but three for their arms. In this manner the entire body is brought into balance.

4. The best training regimen calls for exercising the entire body three or four times a week, always finishing with abdominal exercises. For those intending to train more often, I've designed programs for working half the body on one day and the other half on the next, with stomach exercises done on both days. This means it takes two days to train the entire body. Using this split routine, you will find more exercises for each body part and muscle group, making it easier to get into shape.

5. Work out whenever possible, even if only once a week. Many men interrupt their training due to the press of business, vacations, or travel. They promise themselves they will start training again when they have time. But a few days stretch into a week, and a week stretches into a month as they make one excuse after another, finally losing the habit of training regularly and stopping training altogether.

It doesn't matter if you miss a workout once or twice, or even for a week or two. When you have the time, do at least one workout a week; it will still be beneficial. In this book I have included training programs that can easily be maintained anywhere. If you are forced to skip a full month, be aware that true self-discipline lies in picking up where you left off. There is no point in waiting for a perfect time, because perfect moments are even rarer than perfect bodies.

6. Men and women cannot train in the same manner. The male body structure differs from the female, and the male hormonal balance gives men an average of 15 percent body fat as opposed to a woman's average of 25 percent. Therefore, much of their training will be different, done with a differing number of sets, reps, and weights.

For example, men gain fat mostly in the oblique muscle area that crosses the hips, the low back, the sides of the waist, and the front of the stomach. Women, for the most part, gain fat in the upper thighs, the pelvis, and the back of their arms. For these reasons men should use only training programs designed for them.

7. Use the program that feels best for you. Even though certain programs are designated specifically for maintenance, any program that you find suitable can serve the same purpose. Just train fast and aggressively for one hour, three times a week on alternate days.

Three

Basic Exercise Programs

As in any endeavor, the approach you take to reaching your goals depends on what you start with. In any shape-up plan, therefore, your training program will depend on some fundamental facts about your body—whether you need to lose weight and where, which particular body parts are weak, whether you desire overall muscularity or more specific conditioning, and so on. The five different programs presented in this chapter take into account these considerations among many others that I have encountered in my bodybuilding experience.

One important factor that must be considered is your body type. Although each person will be a combination of three types— *ectomorphic* (thin), *endomorphic* (heavy), and *mesomorphic* (muscular)—one trait is often more dominant than the rest.

Body Types

Ectomorphs, slim and linear with long muscles, usually have long arms and legs. Due to the length of their muscles, they should always do stretching exercises to warm up thoroughly before each training session. Since their goal is directed to gaining muscle size and strength, they should do sets with weights heavy enough to allow only the recommended number of repetitions. If the exercises can be done too easily, more weight should be added. To achieve proportion, ectomorphs must work particularly on their arms and legs, remembering that patience will pay off even if progress seems slow at first.

Ectomorphs should supplement their training with a diet high in protein and with added natural carbohydrates.

Endomorphs tend to become overweight more easily than other body types because their metabolism is usually slow. To achieve maximum results this type of person should use lighter weights and do a higher number of repetitions to burn off fat deposits before building muscle. The weights should be light enough to allow you to do the suggested number of repetitions, taking no more than 60 seconds to rest between sets. Endomorphs should severely limit their intake of fat and should also take care not to consume too many natural carbohydrates.

Mesomorphs are more naturally muscular, with a good skeletal structure similar to mine. Therefore, they usually adapt easily to the discipline of a training program. They should work with heavy weights and do a medium number of repetitions for each exercise. The diet of mesomorphs should be balanced with protein, fat, and carbohydrates.

Since every muscle is a different size, certain muscles will develop more easily than others. Some will require more sets, heavier weights, and fewer repetitions; others will need lighter weights and more repetitions. You will discover this by trial and error based on the individuality of your body type. It is helpful to notice which muscles become sore during training because it is a sign that your program is really working. On the other hand, if something hurts, stop training at once and rest.

Adopting the Basic Programs

Start with any of five programs on pages 50–83 after assessing your body type and goals. If you have not been exercising regularly, Programs 1 or 2 will effect a smooth transition to any of the weight training programs that follow. Anyone with a diagnosed heart condition, high blood pressure, or other medical problems should see a doctor before starting these programs or any type of exercise.

The basic programs should take approximately 10–15 minutes each. Whichever one you choose, be sure to do the exercise in the sequence given, for significant results depend on exercising the body according to its anatomical structure. Certain muscles need to be warmed up before engaging others. If some exercises seem difficult or tiring, do not avoid them, though you may be unable to do the suggested number of sets and reps at the beginning. After a week or two your muscles will adapt to the new demands on them and become stronger.

References to the number of times an exercise is performed are given in terms of sets and reps (repetitions). For example, "1 × 25" noted after Bent-Leg Sit-Up means that you do one set of 25 repetitions, or repeating the exercise 25 times. In Program 4 the number of sets and reps is increased to "2 × 25" for the Bent-Leg Sit-Up. In other words, the exercise is done 25 times before stopping to rest and then another 25 times for a total of 50 repetitions.

All five programs can easily be done at home with the assurance of getting the best possible workout in the shortest amount of time. A pair of dumbbells is required for Programs 1–4. Barbells are also needed for Program 5.

Set reasonable goals, remembering to consider your body's basic structure. The best way to check progress is to take body measurements before beginning the program and after following it for two weeks. Afterwards, keep a record of your progress by measuring yourself periodically. To supplement these tape-measured results, have a friend take a picture of you before starting a program and every few weeks thereafter. Seeing results from both sources, and feeling your clothes fit differently, will provide the motivation needed to reach your goals.

Training Programs

Before you choose a program it is wise to read through the descriptions of all five of them. But to get you started in the right direction, the following list summarizes the differences among the programs.

Program 1 is designed for those who are overweight and have fat deposits around the waist, stomach, and hips. Included are a limited number of exercises for the upper body and legs.

Program 2 puts more emphasis on the upper body and legs and the stomach, hips, and thighs. It is an excellent program for the businessman on the road with suggestions on how to improvise on exercise equipment.

Program 3 exercises the entire body in equal proportion.

Program 4 can be used either by the underweight or by the overweight mesomorphic or ectomorphic body type with different repetitions and sets for each. This program also exercises the entire body.

Program 5 is targeted for those wanting to gain overall muscularity. These exercises also may be used either by the underweight or by the overweight endomorphic body type.

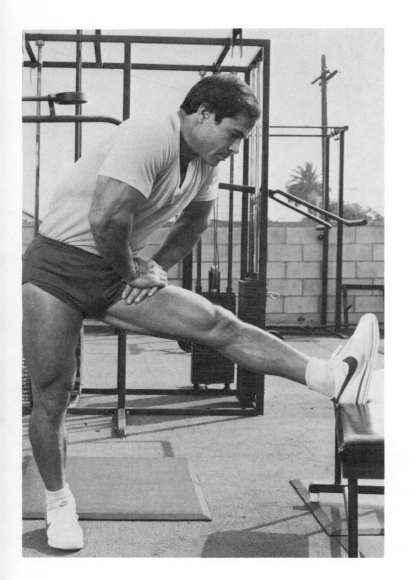

Program #1

Stretching exercises develop the flexibility to reach, bend, and twist and also to maintain a relaxed and balanced body alignment. Although you may have lost suppleness by habitually using only part of your muscles, it can be regained through stretching exercises that progressively elongate the muscle-tendon structures of the body.

Taking only 10 minutes a day, these exercises are done by stretching slowly as far as possible, then stretching a bit more with each repetition. Do not force the movement. Try to relax, breathing evenly and keeping the movement under control. Since elongating the tendons is the purpose of these exercises, do not use bouncing motions that set off reflexes that cause muscles to contract. They should be done continuously, without stopping to rest between exercises.

You will find these exercises easy to do at home, at the office, or in a hotel room. In addition to developing flexibility, you will also alleviate low back problems caused by long hours of sitting at a desk, slumped on a couch, or driving a car.

Standing Hamstring Stretch

Stand with one foot on the edge of a chair, the heel pointing downward. Keeping both legs straight, reach forward until you feel a good stretch along the back of your leg. Hold a moment, keeping the spine as straight as possible to promote increased motion in the lower back. Perform this exercise slowly without forcing the stretch.

1 × 10 on each side

Standing Side Bend

Stand with hands on hips and feet spread far apart. Alternate bending slowly from right to left, each time holding the position for a moment. This will exercise and stretch the oblique muscles and hips.

1 × 10 on each side

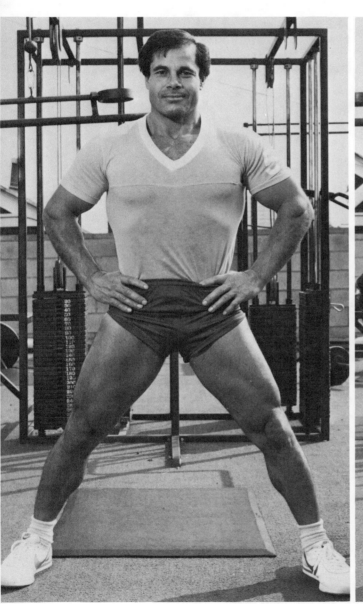
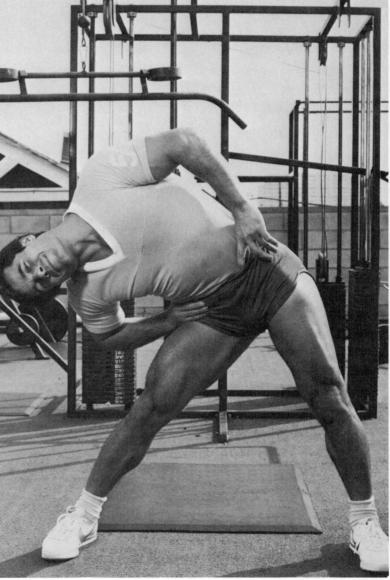

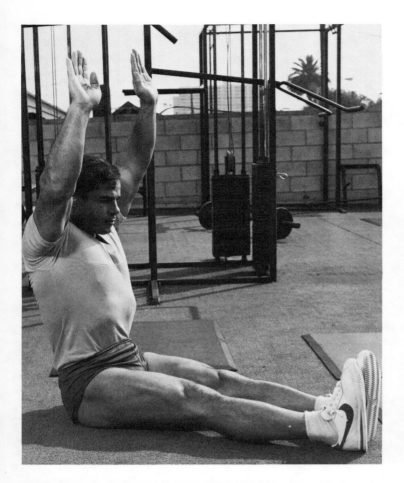

Seated Hamstring Stretch

Sit on the floor with both legs straight out together, toes curved toward the upper body. Slowly reach forward as far as you can without bending the knees. Hold the tips of your toes for 5–10 seconds. Slowly return to the starting position.

1 × 5

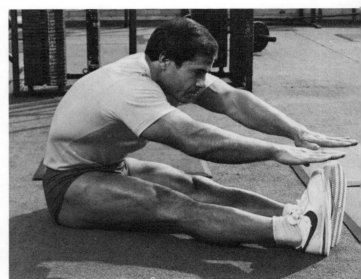

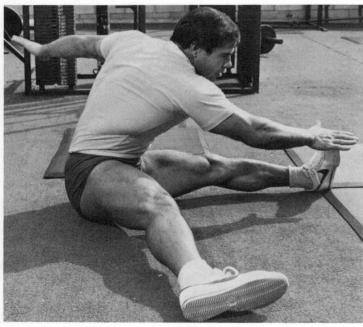

Seated Stretch

Sit on the floor with legs spread wide and knees held straight. Stretch the right hand to the left foot, and then the left hand to the right foot, alternating between them at a fast pace. This will stretch the hamstring, gluteus, and low back muscles.

1 × 7 **on each side**

Knee to Elbow

Lie on your back on the floor with both hands clasped behind your head. Bending one leg at a time, and raising the neck and head from the floor, bring the opposite knee and elbow together. This will firm and tone the stomach with emphasis on the lower section.

1 × 10 on each side

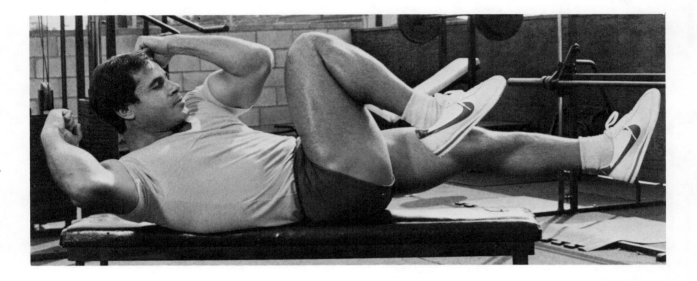

Bent-Leg Sit-Up

Lie comfortably on your back, holding your hands directly over, not behind, your head. Bring the knees toward the chest, trying to bring them to your elbows. Be careful not to raise the low back off the floor to avoid straining it. This exercise firms and strengthens both upper and lower sections of the stomach.

1 × 25

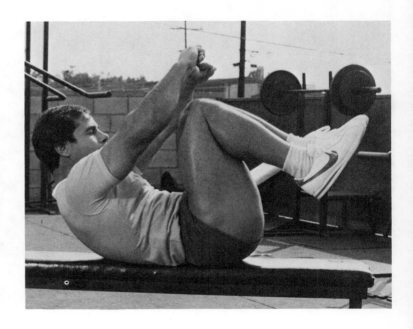

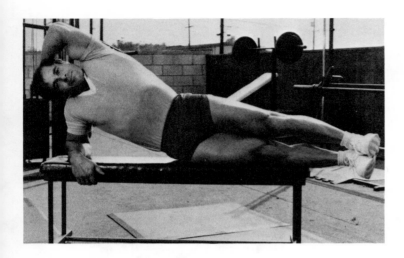

Side Leg Raise

Lie on one side, supported by your elbow. Keeping the upper leg straight, bend the other for a base of support as shown in the photo. Raise and lower the upper arm and leg at the same time. These leg raises are highly effective for reducing fat on the sides of the hips and in the oblique area, better known as the "spare tire." Since they are easier than most exercises, increase the number of repetitions after five days.

1 × 25 on each side
1 × 50 on each side after five days

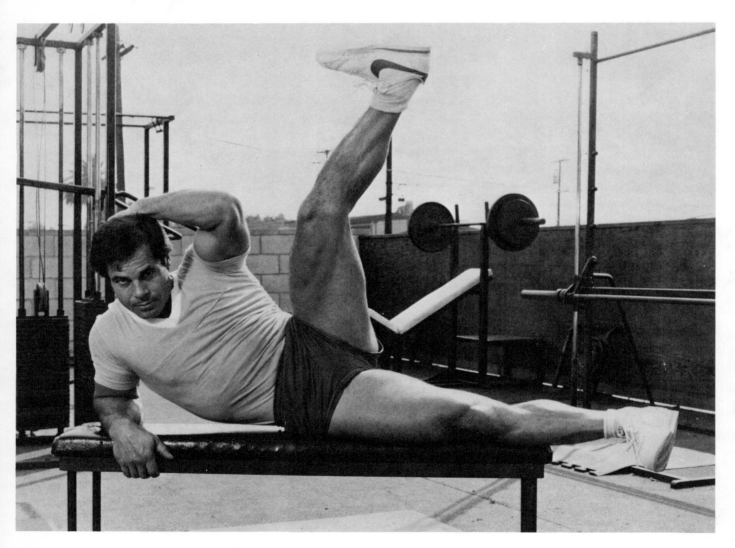

Program #2

Designed to shape up the entire body, this program is easy to maintain when traveling for business or away on vacation. No gym equipment is necessary to do the nine exercises developed to strengthen muscles and reduce fat deposits over the entire body. Particular emphasis is placed on exercises that tighten the abdominal muscles and condition the hip and thigh areas.

Since this program is not geared to development of muscular potential, those concerned with becoming another Hercules can relax. Muscles grow bigger only when forced to put forth additional energy as required in lifting weights.

These exercises take approximately 10–15 minutes to complete.

Standing Side Bend

Stand with hands on hips and feet spread far apart. Alternate bending sideways from right to left. This exercises the oblique muscles and hips.

1 × 10 on each side

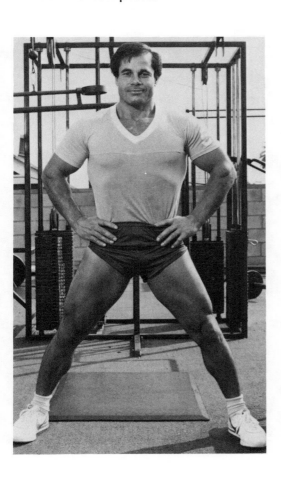
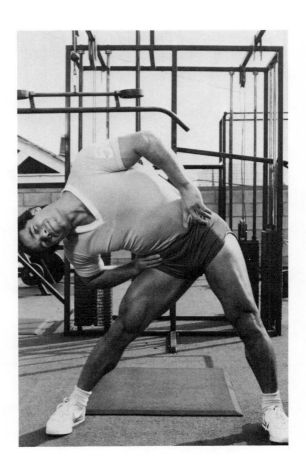

Backhand Stretch

Stand on your toes with the arms raised to just below shoulder level. Leading with the elbow, snap your arms backward as far as possible. This stretches and tones the pectoral muscles.

1 × 10

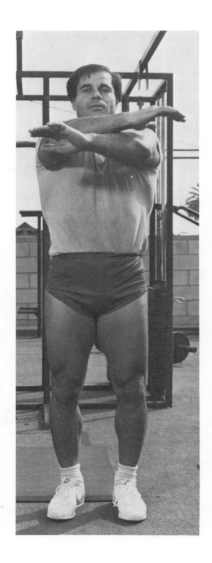
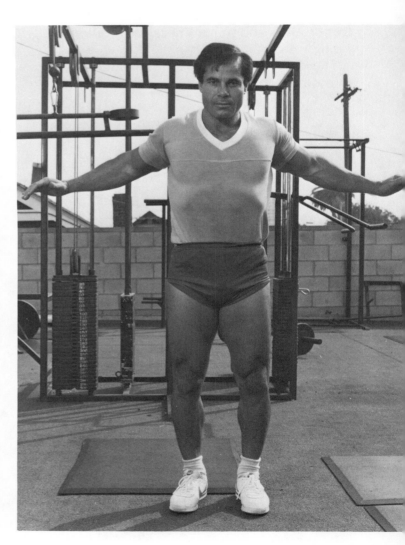

Push-Up Using Chairs

Place two chairs about 24 inches apart. Position yourself as depicted in the photos with each hand on a chair. Push your entire body weight slowly up and down, trying for a complete range of motion. Build up to the required number of repetitions.

3 × 8

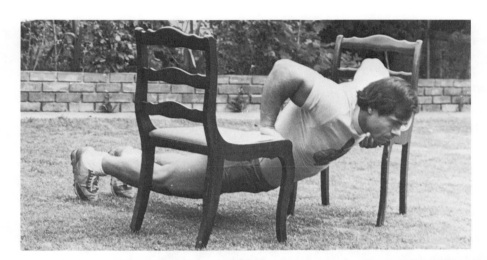

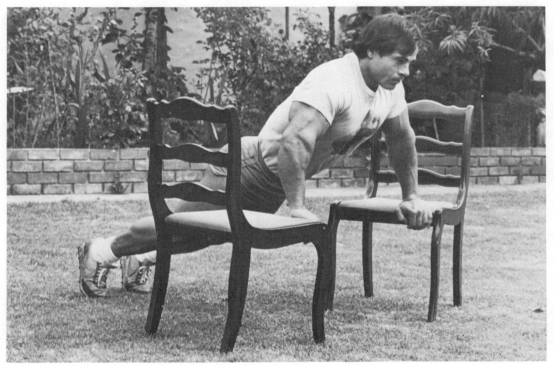

Knee to Elbow

Lie on your back on the floor with both hands clasped behind your head. Raising the neck and head from the floor and bending one leg at a time, bring the opposite knee and elbow together. This firms and tones the stomach with emphasis on the lower section.

1 × 10 on each side

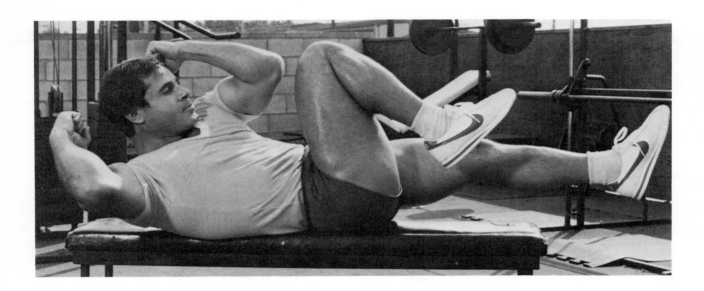

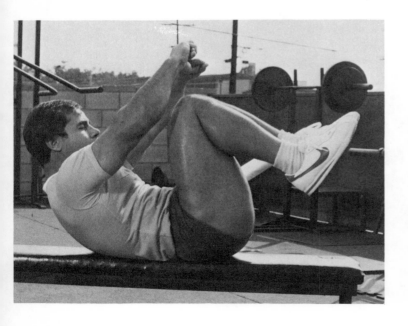

Bent-Leg Sit-Up

Lie comfortably on your back, holding your hands directly over, not behind, the head. Bend the knees toward your chest, trying to bring them to your elbows. Be careful not to raise the low back off the floor to avoid straining it. This firms and strengthens both upper and lower sections of the stomach.

1 × 25

Side Leg Raise

Lie on one side, supported by your elbow. Keeping the upper leg straight, bend the other for a base of support. Raise and lower the upper arm and leg at the same time. Doing these reduces fat on the side of the hips and oblique area. They should be done as quickly as possible.

1 × 25 on each side

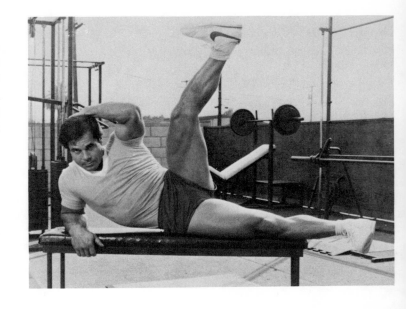

Donkey Kick

Get on your hands and knees, bending the elbows slightly for leverage. Keeping one leg straight, raise it up as high as possible and then lower it while contracting the buttocks. This firms, tones, and reduces fat deposits on the buttocks and backs of the thighs.

1 × 20 on each leg

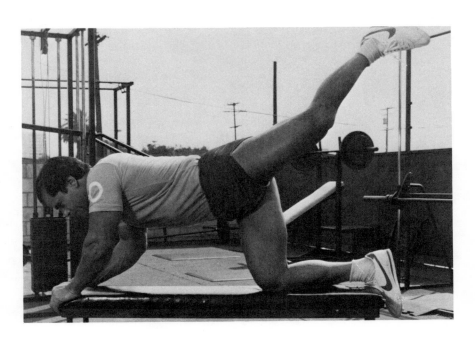

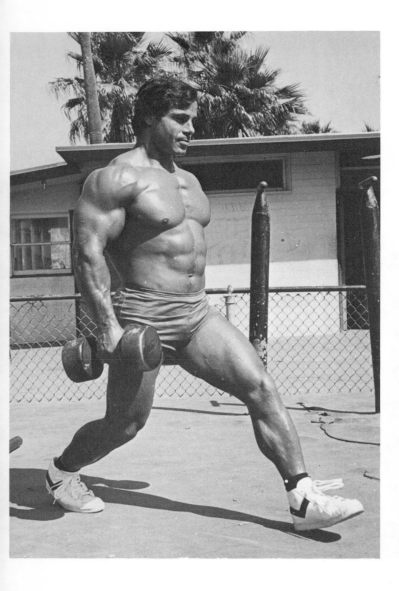

Lunge

Stand erect, holding a book or weight in each hand. Step forward as far as possible with your left foot, lowering your body until the right knee almost touches the floor. Step back and repeat the lunge, starting with the right foot. This will stretch the leg muscles and firm the thighs.

1 × 12 on each leg (first two weeks)
2 × 12 on each leg (thereafter)

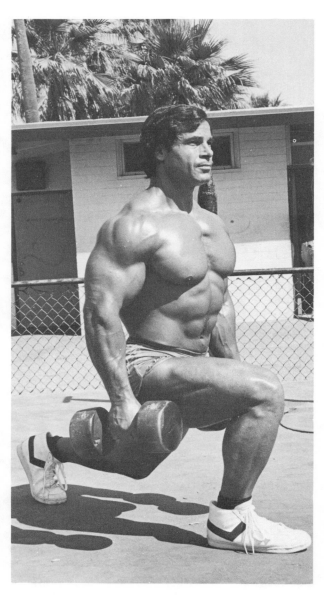

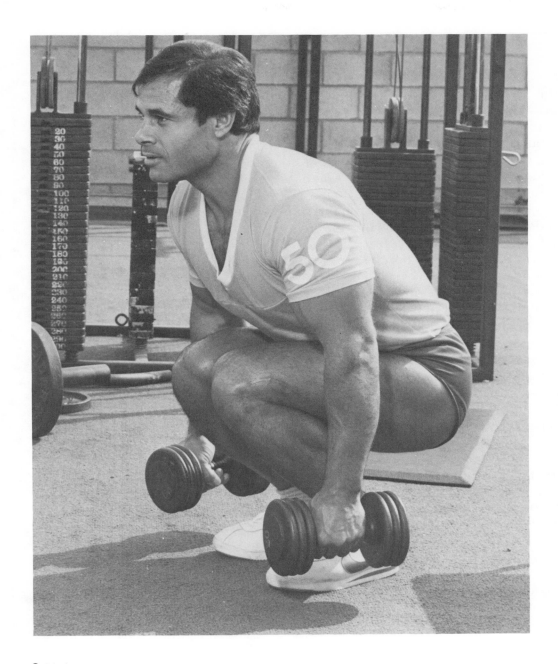

Squat

Stand with heels placed on a block of wood or on a two-inch-thick telephone book. Slowly bend down into a full squat, keeping control of the movement. Slowly stand. This develops endurance and stamina and strengthens the thighs.

1 × 25

Program #3

Beginning with this program you will use a pair of 10- to 15-pound dumbbells. However, if your strength is sufficient to handle heavier weights, use 20-pound dumbbells. Do not swing the weights when raising them. Lift slowly, concentrating on form and focusing attention on the muscles or muscle groups being exercised. Because lowering the weights is easy, there is a tendency to drop them fast instead of keeping the entire movement under control. Aim for smoothness and coordination, and lower the weights slowly to a count of four. At all times, remember to exhale at the moment of exertion (lifting) and inhale as the weights are lowered.

This routine will shape the entire body in proportion, bringing opposing sets of muscles into balance. Muscular potential is developed when you begin forcing muscles to work hard against resistance provided by heavier weights.

These 10 exercises set the foundation for the more advanced programs that follow and build the power, speed, and agility needed for any sport. In total, the benefits gained from this program will equal those of working out in a gym.

Following this program you should rest for 30–60 seconds between sets of exercises and complete the program in about 15–20 minutes.

Hamstring Stretch

Stand with one foot on the edge of a chair, the heel pointing downward. Keeping both legs straight, reach forward until you feel a good stretch along the back of your leg. Hold this position a moment, keeping the spine as straight as possible to promote increased motion in the lower back. Perform this movement slowly without forcing the stretch.

1 × 10 on each leg

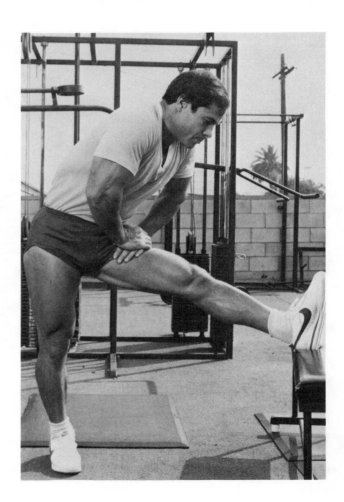

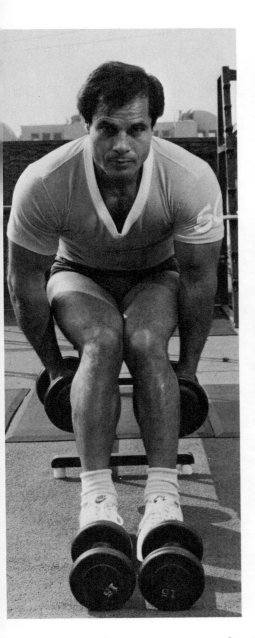
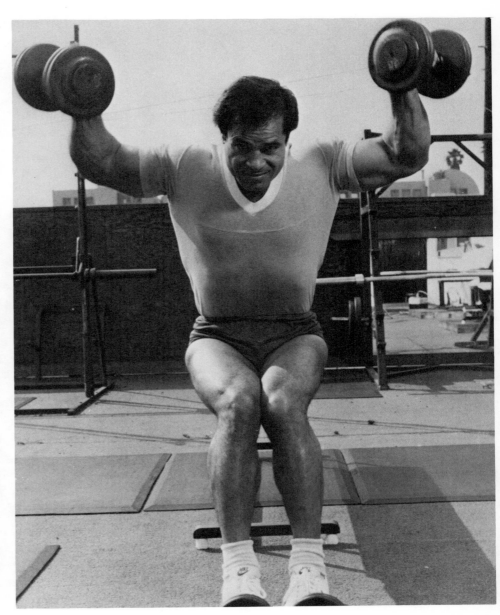

Seated Bent-Over Lateral Raise

Sit on the edge of a chair with your knees slightly bent. Start with the upper body bent over approximately 30–40 degrees. Keeping your elbows bent, lift the dumbbells laterally as high as you can. This movement is felt in the rhomboideus muscles and the backs of the deltoids.

2 × 20   5–10 pounds per dumbbell

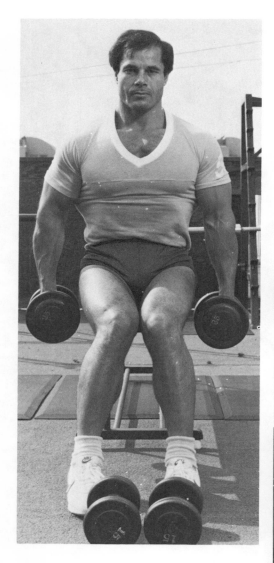

Seated or Standing Lateral Raise

Hold a dumbbell in each hand and stand with feet 12 inches apart or sit on a bench. Bending the elbows slightly, raise the dumbbells slightly higher than shoulder level. This develops the entire deltoid muscle mass, which visually broadens the shoulders.

2 × 20   **5–10 pounds per dumbbell**

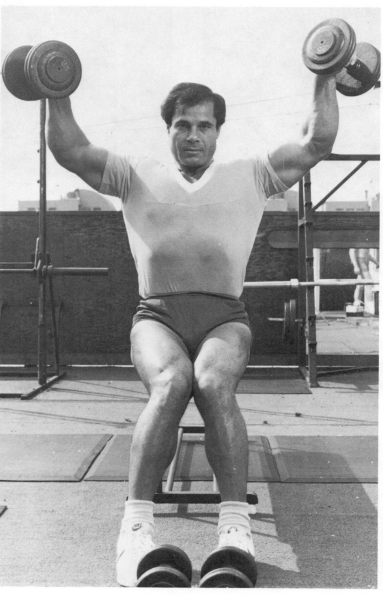

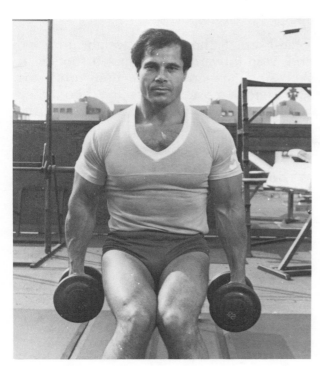

Seated Dumbbell Curl

Sit on a chair holding a dumbbell in each hand. Curl the dumbbells up toward your shoulders and then down again, turning your wrists outward during the curl. Since you can see the bicep muscles move while working, this exercise is excellent for concentrating on muscular movement.

2 × 20   5–10 pounds per dumbbell

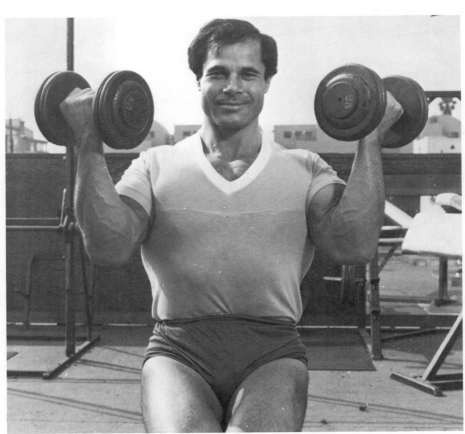

Donkey Kick

Get on your hands and knees, bending the elbows slightly for leverage. Keeping one leg straight, raise it as high as possible and then lower it while contracting the buttocks. This firms, tones, and reduces fat deposits on the buttocks and backs of the thighs.

1 × 20 on each leg

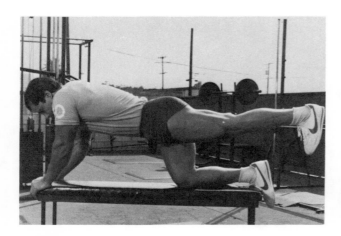

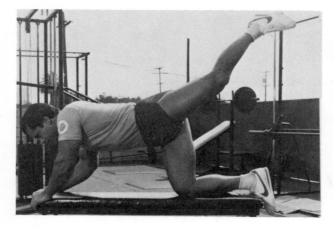

Lunge

Stand erect, holding a weight in each hand. Step forward with your left foot as far as possible, lowering your body until the right knee almost touches the floor. Step back and repeat the lunge, starting with the right foot. This is important for stretching leg muscles and firming thighs.

1 × 12 on each leg (first two weeks)
2 × 12 on each leg (thereafter)

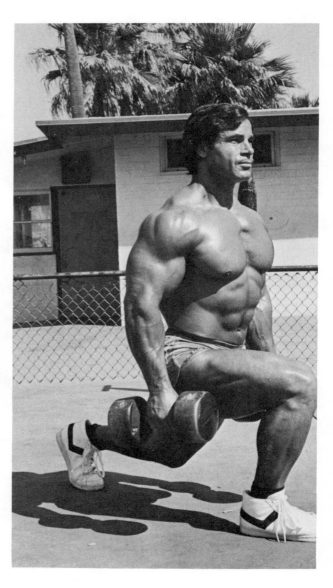

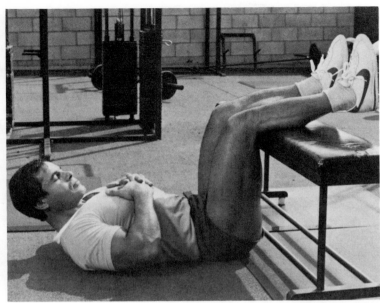

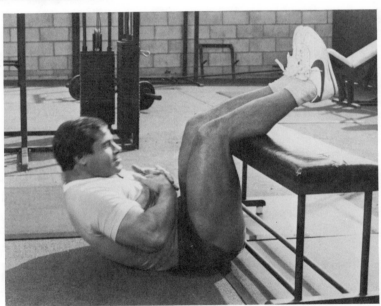

Crunch Sit-Up

Lie comfortably on your back on the floor with your lower legs lying on top of a bench or chair. Keep the knees bent. Clasping your hands over your chest, raise the upper body close to the knees. This works the abdominal muscles, strengthening and tightening them.

3 × 25

Bent-Leg Sit-Up

Lie comfortably on your back, holding your hands directly over, not locked behind, the head. Bend the knees toward your chest, trying to bring them to the elbows. Be careful not to raise the lower back off the floor to prevent straining it. This firms and strengthens both upper and lower sections of the stomach.

1 × 25

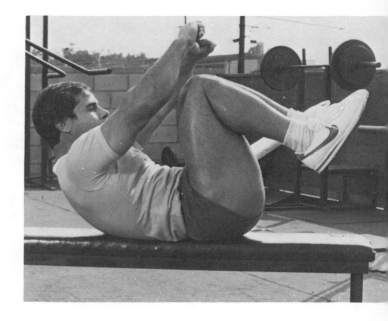

Side Leg Raise

Lie on one side, supported by your elbow. Keeping the upper leg straight, bend the other for a base of support. Raise and lower the upper arm and leg at the same time. These exercises reduce fat on the side of the hips and oblique area. They should be done as quickly as possible.

1 × 25 on each side

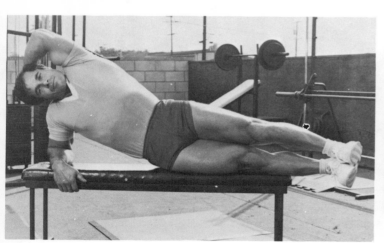

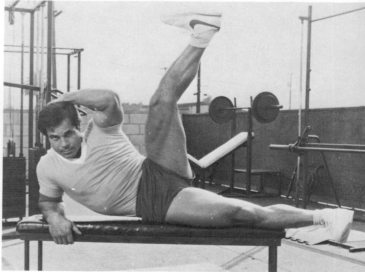

Seated Stretch

Sit on the floor with legs spread as far apart as possible. Alternating between right and left, and keeping your legs straight, stretch your right hand to the left foot and the left hand to the right foot. This stretches the legs, particularly the back of the thighs and lower spine.

1 × 10

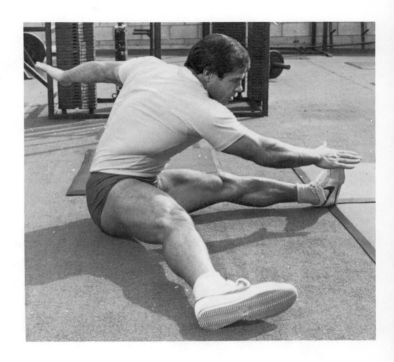

Program #4

At my clinic I design a wide variety of programs for many types of people. Some need to gain or lose weight; others need corrective exercises for spinal problems or injuries sustained in accidents or sports. After checking their body for structural imbalances I ask what they expect to achieve and then tailor individual programs to meet their specific needs.

A great majority of them have the common problem of being either underweight or overweight. Unfortunately, many health club instructors tend to disregard the difference between needing to gain weight and needing to lose it and give the same training program to both types of people.

The key to devising a successful exercise program for both the underweight and the overweight lies in varying the amount of weight used and the number of repetitions. As a general rule, underweight individuals should always use weights heavy enough to allow only 8–10 repetitions. On the contrary, those wanting to lose weight particularly quickly should use very light weights, doing 20–30 repetitions for each exercise. In this way less muscle growth is stimulated and fat deposits are more quickly burned off.

This program is designed for both the underweight and the overweight, since both need to exercise the same muscles and groups of muscles. However, note the change in repetitions. To get the best results from this program, train three times a week, either on Monday, Wednesday, and Friday or on Tuesday, Thursday, and Saturday. Do not train three days in succession because your body will need one day of rest between workouts. Try doing the exercises aggressively and as fast as possible, stopping for no more than one minute between sets. You should complete the program in about 40 minutes.

This routine is ideal for training with a partner even if your weight problems differ.

Bench Press

Lie on a bench (if you don't have upright hooks to support the barbell, hold it across your legs as you lie down). Start by moving the barbell into an upright position over your head. Maintain a grip 30–40 inches wide and lower the barbell, keeping it level across the chest. Inhale while lowering; exhale on the push-up. Keep your spine straight throughout the exercise. This will develop and strengthen the entire chest.

Underweight: 2 × 10
Overweight: 2 × 25   **40 pounds**

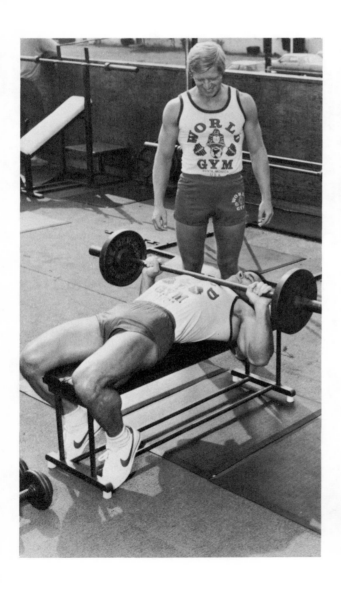
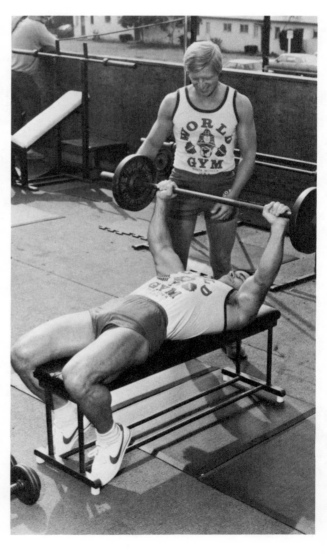

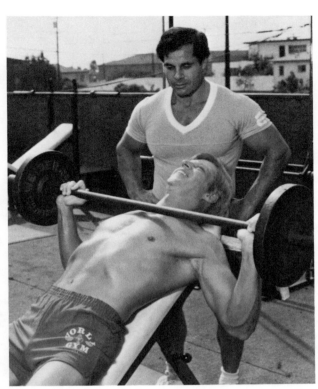

Incline Bench Press

With your back supported by an incline bench, start with the bar held over the eyes. Inhaling deeply, lower it to just below the neck. Exhale when pushing the bar back to the starting position. These bench raises develop and work the muscles of the upper chest.

Underweight: 2 × 10
Overweight: 2 × 25   **40 pounds**

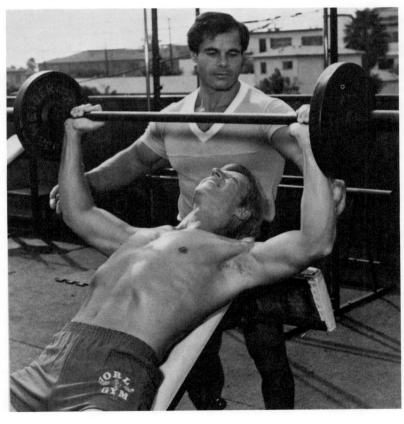

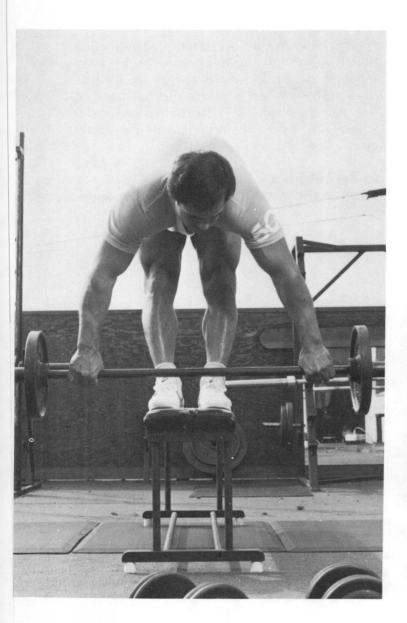
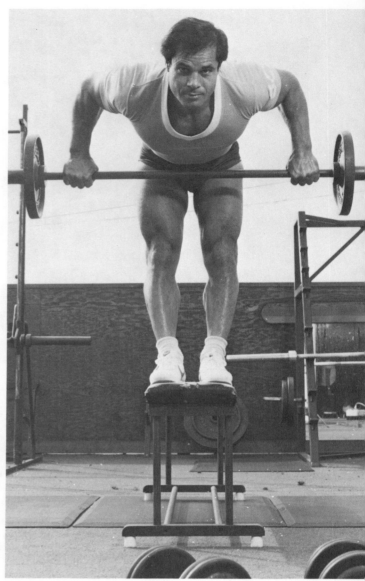

Barbell Rowing

Bend forward from the waist and grasp the bar using a medium grip with palms held down. Bring the bar up to your chest, then lower it. Do not jerk the bar; keep the movement smooth and coordinated. This exercise strengthens the back muscles.

Underweight: 2 × 8
Overweight: 2 × 15   **40 pounds**

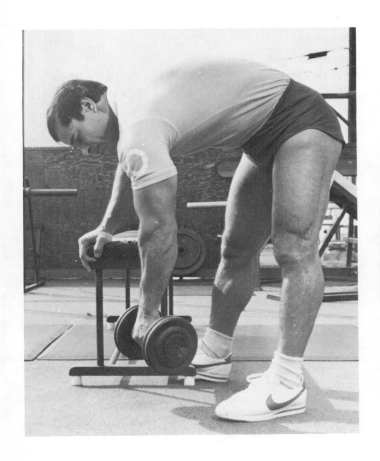
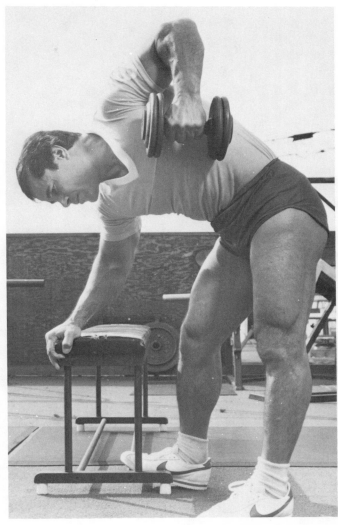

One-Arm Rowing

Stand with the legs apart and the upper body parallel with the floor. Start with the dumbbell held just above the floor between your legs. Pull the dumbbell up, touching the side of your pectoral muscle, then lower it for a complete stretch. Do this movement at a rapid pace. One-Arm Rowing exercises the back muscles from a different angle than the Barbell Rowing.

Underweight: 2 × 8 on each arm
Overweight: 2 × 15 on each arm   30 pounds

Seated Bent-Over Lateral Raise

Sit on the edge of a chair with your knees slightly bent. Start with the upper body bent forward 30–40 degrees. Keeping the elbows bent, lift the dumbbells laterally as high as you can. This should be felt in the rhomboideus muscles and the backs of the deltoids.

Underweight: 2 × 10
Overweight: 2 × 10   **5–10 pounds
per dumbbell**

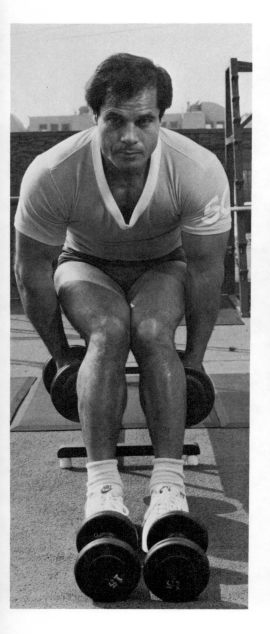

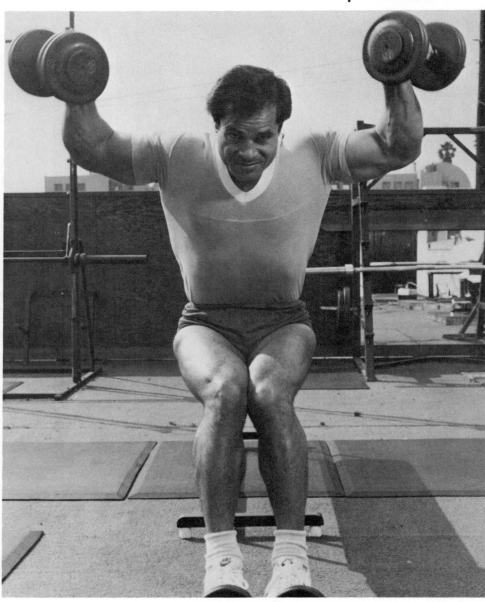

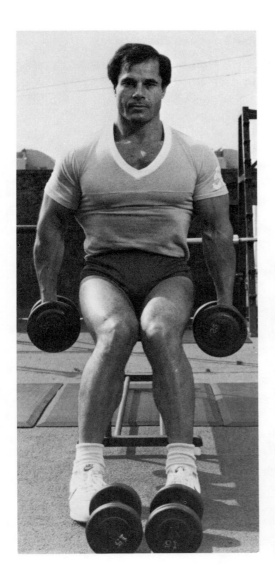

Lateral Raise

Holding a dumbbell in each hand, stand with feet about 12 inches apart. Bend the elbows slightly and raise the dumbbells a little higher than shoulder level. This develops the entire deltoid muscle mass, which visually broadens the shoulders.

Underweight: 2 × 10
Overweight: 2 × 10   **5–10 pounds
                                            per dumbbell**

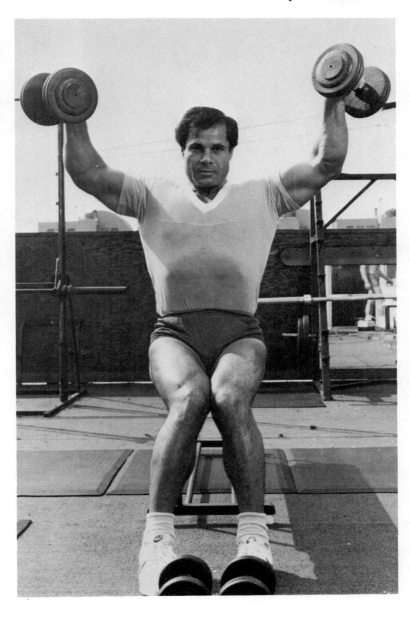

Lying Barbell Triceps Extension

Lie back on a bench, holding a barbell with elbows pointing up. Lower the bar to your forehead, then raise it again for a complete extension without moving the elbows.

Underweight: 2 × 10
Overweight: 2 × 15   **40 pounds**

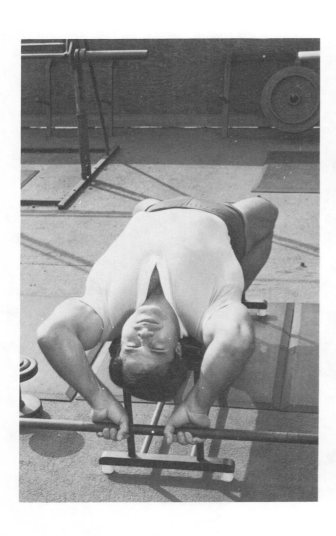
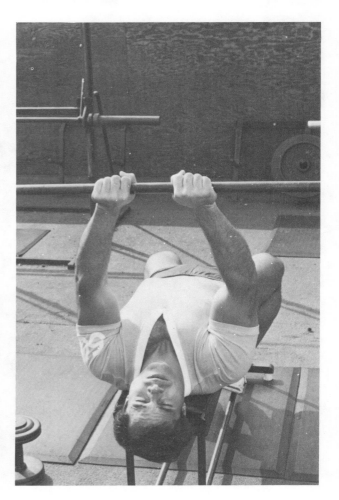

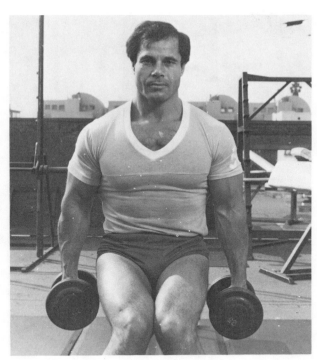

Seated Dumbbell Curl

Sit on a bench, holding a dumbbell in each hand, wrists facing your sides. Curl the dumbbells toward your chest, turning your wrists outward as you curl. You will feel this working the biceps as you curl.

Underweight: 2 × 8
Overweight: 2 × 15
10–20 pounds per dumbbell

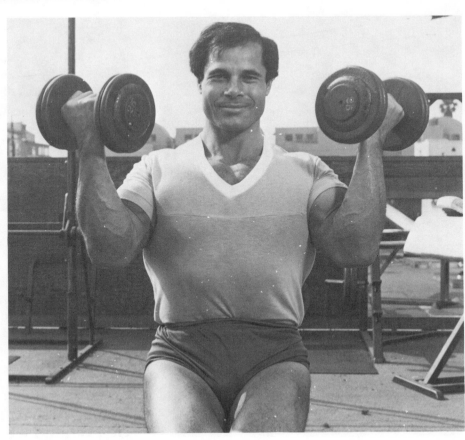

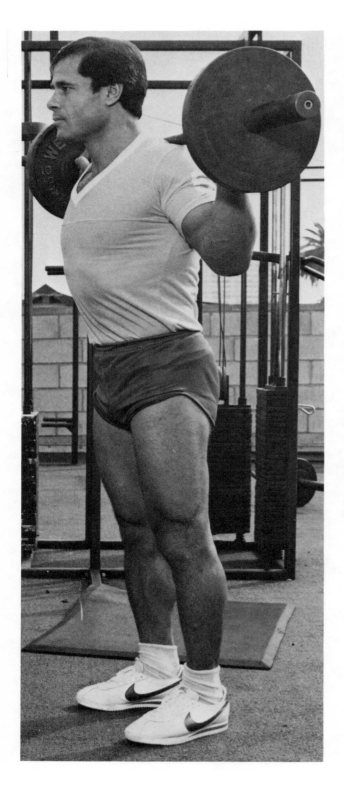

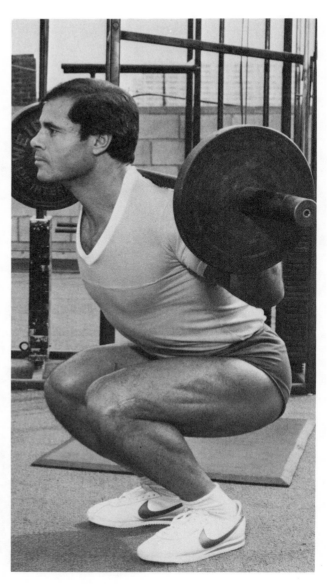

Squat with Bar on Shoulders

Stand with your heels on a wooden block about 2 inches high, keeping your feet about 12 inches apart. Work with the barbell on your shoulders and lower the body into a full squat. Slowly stand. Throughout the exercise, look straight ahead and control the movement. This will develop and strengthen the thighs.

Underweight: 2 × 10
Overweight: 2 × 25   **30 pounds**

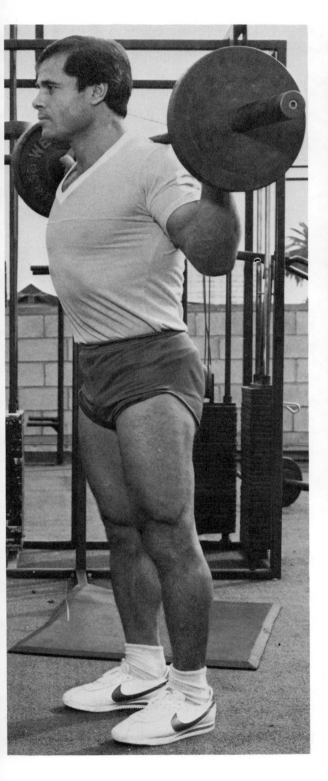

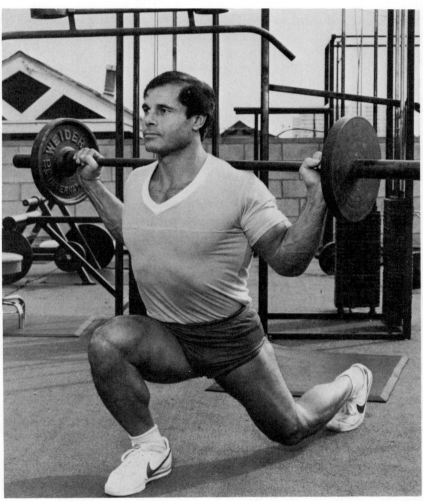

Lunge with Barbell

Stand erect, holding a barbell across your shoulders. Step forward with your left foot as far as possible, lowering your body until the right knee almost brushes the floor. Step back and repeat the lunge starting with the right foot. Hold your head and torso erect. This will stretch the leg muscles and firm the thighs.

Underweight: 2 × 25 on each side
Overweight: 2 × 25 on each side

40 pounds

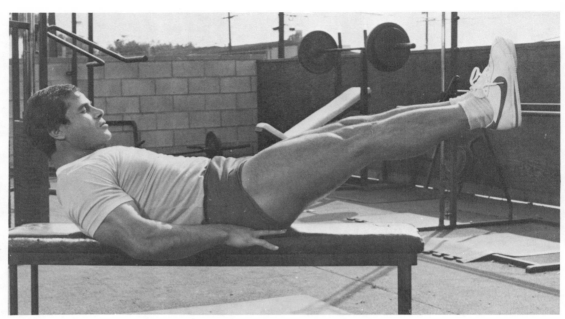

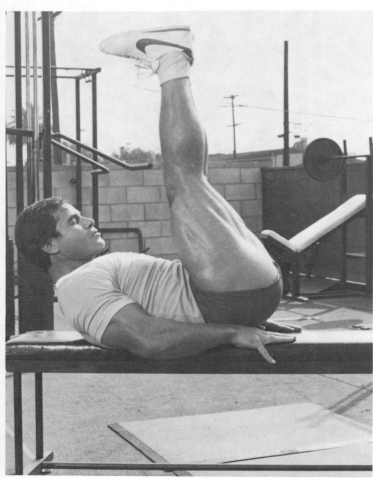

Leg Raise

Lie on your back on the floor or on a bench. Your hands can hang straight down, or they can grip the bench behind your head. Keeping your knees flexed and your toes pointed, raise both legs together straight up. Don't move your hips from the bench.

Underweight: 2 × 25
Overweight: 2 × 25

Bent-Leg Sit-Up

Lie comfortably on your back, holding your hands directly over, not locked behind, the head. Bend the knees toward the chest, trying to bring them to the elbows. Be careful not to raise the lower back off the floor to prevent straining it. This exercise firms and strengthens both upper and lower sections of the stomach.

Underweight: 2 × 25
Overweight: 2 × 25

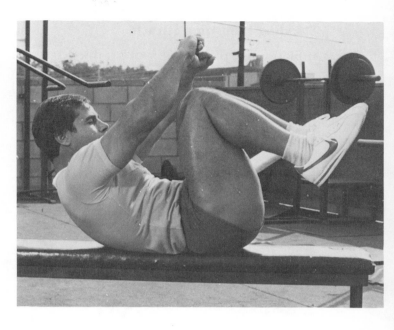

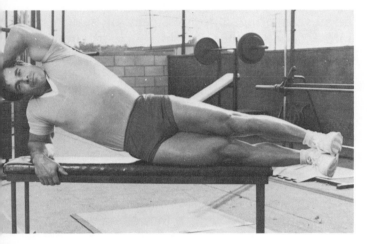

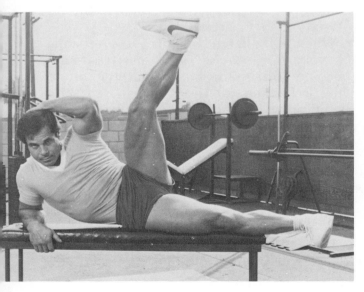

Side Leg Raise

Lie on one side, supported by your elbow. Keeping the upper leg straight, bend the other for a base of support. Raise and lower the upper arm and leg at the same time. This exercise reduces fat on the sides of the hips and oblique area. Do the reps as quickly as possible.

Underweight: 2 × 25 on each leg
Overweight: 2 × 25 on each leg

Standing Hamstring Stretch

Stand and place one foot on the edge of a chair, the heel pointing downward. With both knees straight, bend forward and feel the hamstring muscle stretch along the back of the thigh. Perform this exercise slowly without forcing the stretch.

Underweight: 1 × 10 on each leg
Overweight: 1 × 10 on each leg

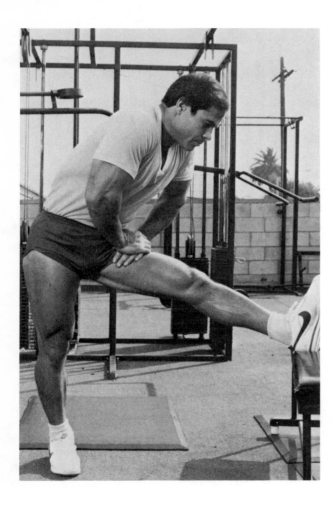

Program #5: Superset Speed Program

Supersetting is a technique for training two muscles or sets of muscles at the same time by alternating between two exercises. The pairs of muscles being worked are antagonistic: as one muscle pulls, the other gives sufficient resistance to balance the pulling muscle. For example, when exercising the upper arms, you will alternate between working the biceps, which flex the elbow, and the triceps, which extend or straighten the arms.

A correct match of muscles being exercised is vital to the supersetting technique because it brings opposing pairs of muscles into balance. Other matches include chest-back, anterior-posterior deltoids, anterior-posterior forearm muscles, and quadriceps-hamstring muscles in the thighs. Because the abdomen cannot be supersetted with another muscle group, it is trained by doing four exercises in rotation: Knee to Elbow, Bent-Leg Sit-Ups, Side Leg Raises, and Crunches.

Throughout this program you will alternate exercises for antagonistic muscles until finished with that body part. In the beginning it may be necessary to reduce slightly the amount of weight used to complete the required number of repetitions.

When using lighter weights and alternating between two exercises, your muscles do not become exhausted; therefore, little or no time is needed for rest between sets. This significantly reduces the amount of time needed for working out. In addition, the continuous high-repetition exercises will reduce fat at a constant rate and increase cardiorespiratory efficiency. When followed in precise sequence, with little or no rest between sets, this program produces highly satisfactory results.

Instructions for performing these exercises can be found in the Glossary.

Exercise 1	Underweight	Overweight
A. Bench Press	2 × 10	2 × 20
B. Barbell Rowing	2 × 10	2 × 20

Exercise 2		
A. Incline Bench Press	2 × 10	2 × 10
B. One-Arm Rowing	2 × 10	2 × 10

Exercise 3		
A. Bent-Over lateral Raise	2 × 8	2 × 15
B. Front Dumbbell Raise	2 × 8	2 × 15

Exercise 4		
A. Lateral Raise	2 × 8	2 × 15
B. Upright Rowing	2 × 8	2 × 15

Exercise 5		
A. Lying Triceps Extension	2 × 8	2 × 15
B. Dumbbell Curl	2 × 8	2 × 15

Exercise 6		
A. Squat	2 × 15	2 × 20
B. Lunge	2 × 15	2 × 20

The next four exercises are done in rotation (i.e., do one set of each before doing the second sets).

Exercise 7		
Knee to Elbow	2 × 25	4 × 25

Exercise 8		
Bent-Leg Sit-Up	2 × 25	4 × 25

Exercise 9		
Side Leg Raise	2 × 25	4 × 25

Exercise 10		
Crunch	2 × 25	4 × 25

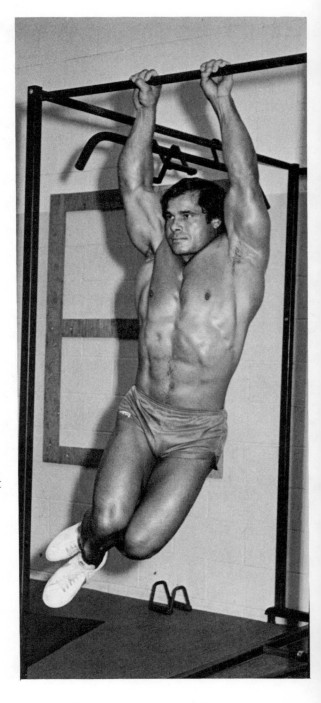

To ease lower back strain by decompressing the spine, hang from a chinning bar, first to the right as shown, then to the left for sixty seconds.

Taking Ten Minutes for an Exercise Break

At the beginning of this century businessmen were not bound to the confines of their offices but traveled on horseback, by stagecoach, and in wagons to reach people now only a phone call away. Our forefathers had no roadside service clubs to repair broken wagon wheels and tow stagecoaches from muddy ditches for them. A hundred times a day their muscles were called on to do work currently done by mechanical devices. Before the machine age more than 50 percent of American males got all the exercise they needed right on the job. Today fewer than ten percent have the benefit of considerable physical activity at work. Some sit, talking on the phone or in conferences, most of the day; others, who work with computer terminals, exercise only their fingers; a great many sit almost immobile as their car moves over city streets, highways, and freeways.

Taking 10 minutes for an exercise break will keep your bodily functions in healthier balance. Effective management of stress is aided by exercise, which acts as a natural tranquilizer in ridding the body of tension. The routine on pages 84–86 will help relieve pent-up stress that might otherwise accumulate during the course of a day.

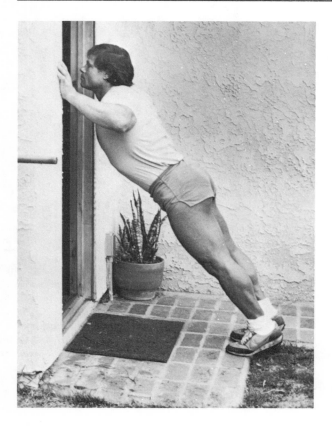

Exercise Break

Wall Push-Up

Standing three to four feet away from the corner of a room, place hands at shoulder height, one on each wall. Holding the body and stomach muscles rigid, slowly move forward, touching your chin to the corner of the wall, then slowly return to starting position.

2 × 10

Push-Up Using Chairs

Place two chairs about 24 inches apart. Position yourself so that each hand is on a chair. Push your entire body weight slowly up and down, trying for a complete range of motion. Build up to the required number of repetitions.

2 × 10

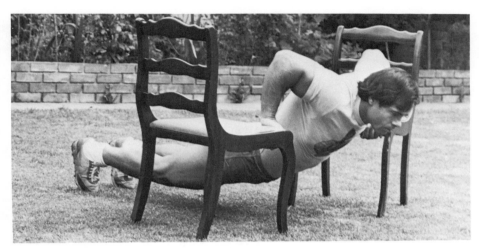

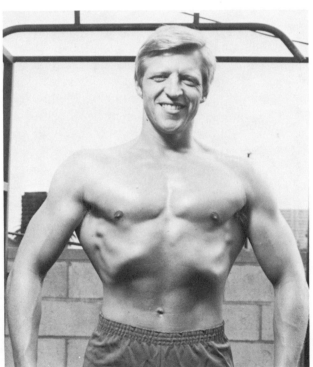

Stand-Up Abdominal

While standing, pull in stomach muscles as hard as possible and hold for six seconds before relaxing.

2 × 10

Seated Leg Raise

While sitting at your desk, raise one leg underneath it, holding the knee straight, until your toes touch the underside of the desk. Try lifting the desk with your leg, keeping your hand on top for stabilization. Hold for six seconds before relaxing.

2 × 10 on each leg

Standing Side Leg Raise

Standing next to your desk for support and leading with your heel, raise one leg to the side as high as possible. Hold for six seconds before returning to starting position.

2 × 10 on each leg

Desk Push-Up

Standing three to four feet away from your desk, place your hands on top of the desk and slowly do a push-up, keeping your back and arms straight.

2 × 10

Four

Advanced Exercise Programs

The exercise programs presented in Chapter 3 can be done at home because they require no special equipment besides weights and a simple bench. The intermediate and advanced programs described in this chapter require equipment best utilized at a gym, or at least require that you have a training partner present to ensure that exercises will be performed safely.

Program #6

This program is designed for training with a partner even if they have different body types. The exercises are the same, but the number of sets and reps differs for the underweight and overweight.

The routine is ideal for use over a long period of time. The first four weeks of doing fewer sets prepare you to carry the full load of exercises.

If you are overweight, use weights light enough to allow you to do the entire number of repetitions for the purpose of burning off fat deposits. The underweight should use weights heavy enough to do only the required number of sets and reps. In

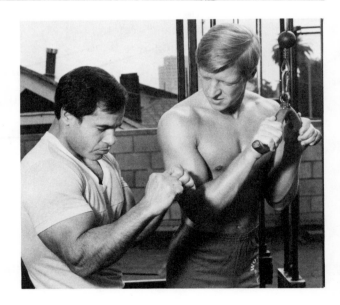

both cases the muscle development takes place over the entire body, except in the stomach and waist areas where the exercises always reduce fat.

You will quickly build up muscles overall by having them gain in size and strength in equal proportions. A balanced body structure will make you look good in clothes. Following this program, you should work out a minimum of three days a week.

Instructions for performing these exercises can be found in the Glossary.

Exercise	Overweight A	Overweight B	Underweight A	Underweight B
Bench Press	2 × 20	3 × 15	2 × 10	3 × 10
Incline Bench	1 × 20	2 × 15	2 × 10	2 × 10
Dip	2 × 5	2 × 10	2 × 10	2 × 10
Pulldown	2 × 20	3 × 20	3 × 10	4 × 10
T-Bar Rowing	1 × 10	2 × 10	2 × 10	3 × 10
Bent-Over Lateral Raise	2 × 10	2 × 10	2 × 8	3 × 8
Lateral Raise	2 × 10	3 × 10	3 × 8	3 × 8
Triceps Pushdown	2 × 20	3 × 12	3 × 10	4 × 8
Lying Triceps Extension	2 × 15	3 × 12	3 × 10	3 × 8
Seated Dumbbell Curl	2 × 10	2 × 10	2 × 10	3 × 8
Preacher Bench Curl	2 × 10	3 × 10	3 × 10	4 × 8
Leg Extension	3 × 25	4 × 25	3 × 20	4 × 20
Leg Curl	2 × 25	3 × 25	3 × 20	3 × 20
Squat	2 × 20	3 × 20	3 × 10	4 × 8
Calf Raise	3 × 20	5 × 20	3 × 15	5 × 15
Bench Leg Raise	3 × 25	4 × 25	3 × 25	3 × 25
Bent-Leg Sit-Up	3 × 25	4 × 25	3 × 25	3 × 25
Side Leg Raise	3 × 50	4 × 50	3 × 50	3 × 50
Back Leg Stretch	1 × 10	1 × 10	1 × 10	1 × 10
Standing Side Bend	1 × 10	1 × 10	1 × 10	1 × 10

Column A: first four weeks
Column B: maintenance and progress

Program #7

Here is another program developed for training partners of different body types. This split routine contains more exercises and sets because the workout is divided between two days. Similar to supersetting, the routine assigns different body parts to separate days with stomach exercises done during each workout. The breakdown of a split routine offers an optimum combination of exercise and rest, since every body part is trained only twice a week, giving muscles additional time to recuperate between sessions.

This is also a long-term program, with the first four weeks forming the foundation for doing the higher number of sets. As in Program #6, muscle strength and development increase overall, and the same rules apply for the amounts of weight used.

Instructions for these exercises are in the Glossary.

MONDAY AND THURSDAY

Exercise	Overweight		Underweight	
	A	B	A	B
Bench Press	2 × 20	3 × 15	2 × 10	4 × 8
Incline Bench Press	1 × 20	2 × 15	2 × 10	2 × 8
Dip	1 × 7	2 × 10	1 × 8	2 × 8
Pulldown	2 × 20	3 × 20	2 × 10	3 × 8
T-Bar Rowing	1 × 10	2 × 10	2 × 10	3 × 8
One-Arm Rowing	1 × 10	1 × 10	1 × 10	2 × 8
Bent-Over Lateral Raise	2 × 10	2 × 10	2 × 10	3 × 8
Lateral Raise	2 × 10	3 × 10	2 × 10	3 × 8
Triceps Pushdown	2 × 10	3 × 15	2 × 10	3 × 8
Lying Triceps Extension	2 × 15	2 × 15	2 × 10	3 × 8
Seated Dumbbell Curl	2 × 10	2 × 10	2 × 10	3 × 8
Preacher Bench Curl	2 × 10	3 × 10	2 × 10	3 × 8
Bench Leg Raise	3 × 25	3 × 25	1 × 20	2 × 25
Side Leg Raise	3 × 50	3 × 50	1 × 50	1 × 50
Back Leg Stretch	1 × 10	1 × 10	1 × 10	1 × 10
Side Bend	1 × 10	1 × 10	1 × 10	1 × 10

Column A: first four weeks
Column B: maintenance and progress

TUESDAY AND FRIDAY

Exercise	Overweight		Underweight	
	A	B	A	B
Leg Extension	3 × 25	4 × 25	3 × 20	4 × 25
Leg Curl	2 × 25	3 × 25	2 × 20	3 × 25
Squat	2 × 20	3 × 20	3 × 10	4 × 8
Calf Raise	3 × 15	5 × 15	4 × 15	6 × 10
Leg Raise	2 × 25	4 × 25	2 × 25	2 × 25
Bent-Leg Sit-Up	2 × 25	4 × 25	2 × 25	2 × 25
Side Leg Raise	2 × 25	4 × 50	2 × 25	2 × 25
Back Leg Stretch	1 × 10	1 × 10	1 × 10	1 × 10

Hand on Chinning Bar for Stretch—1 minute

Column A: first four weeks
Column B: maintenance and progress

Gym Training Program

This program is geared to train the entire body in one day, giving you a choice of going to the gym either two or three times a week. The best possible schedule is to train on Monday, Wednesday, and Friday or on any other three days with one free day between sessions to let the muscles recuperate. This is one of the basic principles of bodybuilding and, if combined with hard training, pushing yourself, and the use of heavy weights, it brings quick results.

The numbers in parentheses following each exercise name is a recommended poundage range (divide by two for dumbbell exercises), but you have to figure out what's best for you. There's really no way to tell you how many pounds to lift for two reasons: (1) each person has a different level of strength, and (2) your strength will increase each week. The only guideline is finding the 10th repetition a struggle but still manageable. If you cannot do 10 reps the weight is too heavy; if they are done easily, the weight is too light.

Although the gym may sometimes be crowded, find a way to train continually rather than waiting between sets of exercises for someone to finish using a piece of equip-ment. Rest periods during the entire workout should run from 30 seconds to one minute, and the stomach exercises should be done with the shortest possible break between sets.

Gym Training Program 1: For the Entire Body

Train two or three days a week.

Exercise	Sets/Reps
Bench Press (80–120)	2 × 10
Incline Bench Press (60–100)	3 × 10
Pulldown (60–100) or Chin	3 × 12
Pulley Rowing (40–80)	3 × 10
Bent-Over Lateral Raise (20–60)	3 × 10
Lateral Raise (10–30 each hand)	3 × 10
Lying Triceps Extension (20–60)	3 × 12
Triceps Pushdown (30–70)	3 × 12
Dumbbell Curl (30–70)	3 × 8
Preacher Bench Barbell Curl (20–60)	3 × 8
Leg Extension (20–60)	3 × 25
Leg Curl (10–50)	3 × 20
Squat (70–120)	2 × 15
Lunge (40–80)	2 × 10
Calf Raise (80–120)	4 × 15
Crunch Sit-Up	3 × 25
Lying Side Leg Raise	3 × 25

Gym Program 2: Split Routine

Targeted for those who want a greater challenge, this advanced program was designed to be used indefinitely. Your training is divided into two-day workouts that exercise the upper part of your body on Monday and Thursday and the lower part on Tuesday and Friday. Your stomach is trained each time you work out, that is, four days a week. Your muscles are given time to rest and recuperate on Wednesday, Saturday, and Sunday.

In some cases the number of sets for a particular body part do not match exactly because most people are stronger in their flexor muscles than in the extensors. For a simple demonstration of the inequality, observe the greater power and flexibility of turning your hand down, as if picking up an object, rather than turning it back toward the wrist. Therefore, the arm exercises include a total of nine sets for the triceps (extensors) and only seven sets for the biceps (flexors).

If done regularly and consistently these exercises will allow you to build muscle mass, just remember to add weight gradually. Also keep in mind that proportion and symmetry are what successful bodybuilding is all about, so be sure to exercise all muscle groups.

Gym Program 2: Split Routine

Train four days a week.

MONDAY AND THURSDAY

Exercise	Sets/Reps
Back Leg Stretch	2 × 10
Side Bend	2 × 20
Bench Press	5 × 10
Incline Bench Press	3 × 10
Dips	3 × 10
Chin in Front of Neck	5 × 10
Barbell or T-Bar Rowing	3 × 10
One-Arm Rowing	2 × 10
Bent-Over Lateral Raise	4 × 10
Lateral Raise with Dumbbells or Cables	4 × 10
Standing Dumbbell Press	2 × 20
Lying Triceps Extension	5 × 12
Triceps Pushdown	4 × 12
Seated Dumbbell Curl	4 × 12
Preacher Bench Curl	3 × 10
Bent-Leg Sit-Up (done in rotation with next three exercises)	4 × 25
Crunch (in rotation)	4 × 25
Leg Raise (in rotation)	4 × 25
Lying Side Leg Raise (in rotation)	4 × 25

TUESDAY AND FRIDAY

Exercise	Sets/Reps
Back Leg Stretch	2 × 10
Side Bend	2 × 20
Lunge (each leg)	3 × 10
Leg Extension	4 × 25
Leg Curl (fewer sets are done for the hamstrings than the quadriceps to help prevent knee (injuries)	2 × 25
Squat (go from light weight to as heavy as you can safely handle)	5 × 10
Calf Raise	7 × 15
Front Calf Raise	5 × 15
Bent-Leg Sit-Up (in rotation)	4 × 25
Crunch (in rotation)	4 × 25
Leg Raise (in rotation)	4 × 25
Lying Side Leg Raise (in rotation)	4 × 25

Five

Nutrition

The body is made up of many materials that must be nourished by a wide variety of foods to ensure the harmonious working of its many parts. Therefore, it is important that your daily decisions regarding nutrition be properly guided rather than conditioned by faddist influences. Great gains can be made toward establishing healthful eating habits if people pay the same attention to the nutritional value of food as they pay to its caloric content. For example, many people know that a medium-sized baked potato has about 100 calories, but very few are aware that it is also rich in minerals such as calcium, magnesium, sulphur, and potassium or that it has about half as much vitamin C as an average tomato and as much thiamin as two slices of whole-grain bread.

Fortunately, the volume and tempo of nutrition research in relation to health have greatly increased during the past 10 years. The results of this research have triggered publication of many books, periodicals, and newsletters, which are rapidly expanding the nutritional knowledge of the general public. While most of the information is excellent, some experts present ideas and diet programs that are conflicting. Their focus is sometimes too narrow, disregarding the fact that the body, broadly speaking, is the product of nutrition and physical activity. My approach to providing nutritional guidelines will differ from that of others due to my early background and the knowledge gained from developing my own body to championship status. In great measure, my tremendous strides in boxing, bodybuilding, and powerlifting are attributable to excellent nutritional practices during the first 19 years of my life when all my food was fresh and organically grown.

The Fundamentals of Nutrition

As previously mentioned, I was born in Sardinia, an Italian island situated 250 miles west of the mainland. One side of the island faces the Tyrrhenian Sea and the coast of Italy; the other overlooks the western Mediterranean and the coast of Spain. Sardinia remains the least spoiled, most naturally beautiful island in the Mediterranean. Strong prevailing winds keep the air fresh, and there is scarcely any industry to produce smog. Most of the inhabitants maintain good health and mental vigor into old age because the majority do hard physical labor, requiring them to work out of doors the entire day. They live frugally but are not oppressed by their poverty since each family has its own land and animals. Surrounded by friends and relatives they have known since childhood, Sardinians enjoy the peace of mind that results from living among those who share the same values and honor the same traditions.

Little that is basic changes in Sardinia. Life remains unhurried, in tune with the elements of nature and the change in seasons. As during my boyhood, the food is grown organically in mineral-rich soil and without chemicals. Gassing tomatoes to make them red and spraying lettuce to keep it fresh for more than a month are totally unknown in Sardinia. Fruits and vegetables are picked only when ripe, and for this reason I find a vast difference in taste between fruits and vegetables in Sardinia and those sold in America markets. My mother rarely purchased anything in a store and never used canned foods. She went directly into the garden, picking vegetables when they were needed to prepare a meal. Nothing was stored.

Because there is little in the way of refrigeration, meat and poultry are eaten fresh. Animals are killed at the right time and never given food, drugs, or hormones to supply a mass market. Meat from older animals is used for soups and a variety of dishes requiring slow simmering with vegetables over a low heat. Younger animals such as lamb are roasted without seasoning over a wood fire in the fireplace. Placed lengthwise on a rough rod like a spit, they are watched and turned constantly, so the meat cooks evenly over the glowing wood and very little smoke is absorbed.

From childhood on I rarely had any candy, sweet pastry, or other products made from refined sugar, which interferes with many normal metabolic processes. My main source of sweets was in the form of fruits and other natural carbohydrates. Although Sardinia is

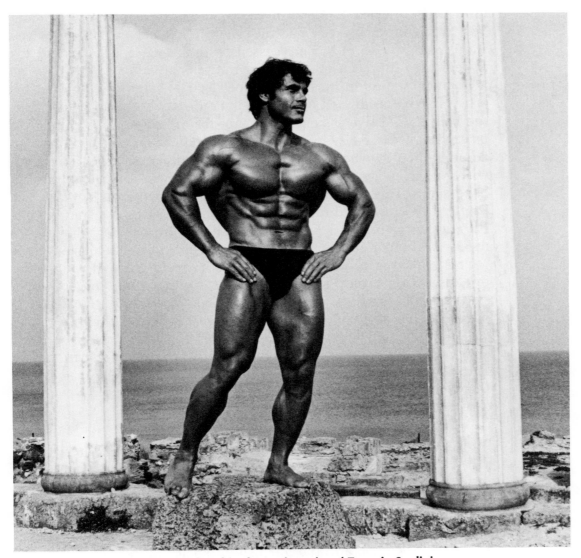

A younger Franco poses on a pedestal in the ancient city of Tarus in Sardinia.

lacking in mechanical luxuries, fruit is abundant. Therefore, I went into the garden every day and ate many different types of fruit, especially grapes, figs, oranges, and apples. Grapes are really a wonder food, very rich in minerals and certain vitamins. I often drink grape juice directly before going to the gym because it is excellent for building energy.

Bad Eating Habits

When I began studying for my PhD in nutrition I was amazed to discover that my people, though poor and simply educated, intuitively knew more about proper eating habits than most well-informed Americans. None of the meals have any empty calories. The Sardinian housewife does not shop in a supermarket; therefore, she is not enticed to buy processed or junk foods packaged for eye appeal with little consideration for nutritional value.

In Sardinia, as in most of Europe, food is eaten in the following order. We begin dinner by having a small bowl of soup, which cues the body's digestive system to prepare for digestion. This is followed by the main course, which provides protein (fish, poultry, or meat) accompanied by whatever vegetable is in season. A large salad made with freshly picked vegetables is eaten afterward. A little later we have some fruit and Sardinian lamb cheese, which is very rich in protein, vitamins, and minerals. Last, but not least, is a small cup of Italian espresso. Good homemade wine is always served with the meals, providing additional minerals and enzymes that aid digestion.

This typical meal seems planned with a careful eye on the digestive processes to prevent nutritional deficiencies caused by improper synthesis of enzymes. By eating protein foods first the digestive juices are not diluted, giving hard-to-digest nutrients the best chance of being fully acted on by gastric enzymes. Pepsin, a protein-splitting enzyme, is the most essential. Secreted by glands lining the upper half of the stomach, it acts best when the gastric juice is acid. For this reason I suggest eating salads either with the protein course or directly afterward.

In Los Angeles and many other American cities the salad is served as an appetizer before the main course. Usually it is covered with a heavy, bottled dressing and accompanied by bread and butter. Most people are under the impression that they will eat less of the main course, which they consider more fattening, if they stuff themselves with bread and salad. I have observed this practice for many years and noticed that the only foods remaining on their plates were the skin of a baked potato, the garnishing sprigs of parsley, and a few limp, overcooked vegetables. Despite their best intentions to cut calories, they were actually eating more and digesting it less. There-fore, it is not surprising that magazines and newspapers run feature articles on diets as regularly as letters to the editor and horoscopes.

The Problem with Calorie Counting

Calorie consciousness has not proved successful in the long run. Adding a column of figures that neatly totals 1,200 calories seems like an efficient, no-nonsense method of harnessing the intake of food; however, most people soon tire of this numbers game and go on eating binges that are even worse than before. In addition, they have acquired the bad habit of saving hundreds of calories to splurge on rich desserts and other foods having little nutritional value. Quite often people say, "There are no calories in this; it won't make me fat." This is not always true. Many unprocessed and unrefined foods high in calories are not fattening provided the body can use them efficiently. On the other hand, many low-calorie items, such as diet drinks, can cause a weight gain. These drinks are loaded with various chemicals (including sodium chloride, which causes water retention). Research has shown that these chemicals place a strain on the thyroid gland, altering regulation of the metabolic rate, which actually causes weight reduction to be more difficult! This is just one example of how "dieting" to lose weight can be self-defeating.

Any diet should be as simple and natural as possible with all things in moderation—protein, fat, and unrefined carbohydrates. Instead of overloading yourself at one meal, have several small meals a day. Eat only when physically hungry and not to compensate for frustration, anxiety, stress, or emotional upheavals. Too often food is used as a tranquilizer when intense physical activity would serve the same purpose of alleviating tension. Having moods rather than appetite dictate eating habits is one of the major reasons for overeating and finding it difficult to maintain a nutritionally balanced diet.

Allergies

It is also necessary to consider that certain foods may not be good for you, even though they are of high nutritional value. It is often said, "One man's meat is another man's poison." Therefore, keep in mind that your family and friends may have no problem digesting foods that give you allergic reactions.

At our clinic we are currently involved with several doctors working on allergy testing. In evaluating results we are gaining insight into specific foods and chemicals that damage the body by placing it under constant stress to combat toxic foods and substances. For example, when the blood tests of 1,000 adult patients were evaluated, we discovered that a majority were allergic to dairy products, though their nutritional value is first rate. Milk and cheese are high in vitamin A and calcium, and yogurt helps regulate bacteria in the colon. We all know that babies and young children need milk; serious conditions regarding growth and bone formation will result when too little is consumed.

The reason children thrive on milk while adults suffer allergic reactions is the difference between their digestive processes. The young have an abundance of rennin, an enzyme that curdles the milk so the protein is precipitated and can be acted on by the pepsin found in the upper half of the stomach. Since the production of rennin in adults is limited, dairy products are not properly digested and can cause many problems, ranging from weight gain to headaches or sinus conditions.

Other symptoms of food allergies include depression, loss of energy, rashes, and swelling of hands and feet. Below is a list of the foods causing most people allergic reactions. Using this as a guide, you may become aware of certain food intolerances in your own eating patterns. If so, have a test that measures the morphological changes in your white blood cells as they interact with extracts of these specific foods. When microscopically examined in the laboratory, changes are evident if the food is harmful, but the cells remain intact if not causing allergic reactions.

Allergic/Non-Allergic Food

The following lists will guide you in maintaining an allergen-free diet, but bear in mind that certain items will vary to a degree from individual to individual. Food not shown on either list falls between the two categories.

Allergy-Causing Foods

Animal Foods
- All milk, including low-fat milk, butter, buttermilk, yogurt, whey
- All cheese, including cottage cheese, sour cream
- All salad dressings, including mayonnaise and blue cheese
- Honey
- Bacon, pork, beef, and duck

Plant Foods
- Cocoa, chocolate, cola, nuts, sugar and molasses
- All hard alcohol, corn, white rice, bananas, beans, vanilla

Other Substances
- Most drugs, saccharin, all diet drinks, and food coloring

Allergen-Free Foods

Animal Foods
- Shrimp, crab, lobster, scallops, oysters, tuna, swordfish, shark, trout, sole, snapper, salmon, halibut, bass, cod, catfish, flounder, and caviar
- Turkey, chicken, liver, eggs, veal, and rabbit

Plant Foods
- Lemons, oranges, grapefruit, tangerines, raspberries, boysenberries, blackberries, grapes, pineapple, apples, pears, papaya, and cantaloupe
- Broccoli, cauliflower, Brussels sprouts, cabbage, radishes, mustard, lettuce, artichokes, carrots, mushrooms, asparagus, onions, garlic, potatoes, eggplant, tomatoes, green peppers, spinach, alfalfa, and coffee.

Food Combining

By combining foods properly and keeping meals simple you can avoid many digestive problems and be assured that your body is assimilating and utilizing nutrients efficiently instead of being forced to store them in folds of fat. Before nutrients can enter the blood stream they must undergo chemical changes. Digestive enzymes convert proteins into amino acids, starches and complex sugars into simple sugars, and fat into fatty acids and glycerol. Because each enzyme reacts to a specific class of food, it is important not to combine too many different types at one meal.

Unlike most Europeans, who habitually limit their food combinations because they usually eat only foods that are in season, Americans are accustomed to having a great variety. This was not the case until after World War II, when supermarkets and home freezers entered the American way of life. Today the average refrigerator /freezer has a 17-cubic-foot capacity, allowing for an astonishing variety of foods to be stored and selected. Ready at hand for introduction to any meal are soda pop, breads and buns, an array of salad dressings, desserts, frozen fruits and vegetables. No matter the season, strawberries, frozen fast in sugared syrup and chemicals, are ready to be defrosted and combined with a mound of canned whipped cream to top off a meal. It is bad enough that frozen and canned foods are of dubious nutritional value, but the practice of choosing from a number of foods due to their immediate availability has led many Americans away from a natural way of eating and combining foods.

When you eat food the body can use efficiently, it will not show up as a weight increase. Consider protein foods as fuel that is either used by the body when eaten or thrown off as waste if the body is adequately nourished and does not need it. Since the stomach secretes a different kind of enzyme during the digestion of proteins, carbohydrates and protein food should be eaten separately as much as possible. For this reason I recommend not combining several proteins in the same meal because the stomach will release different enzymes, making digestion more difficult.

In general, it is best to eat either vegetables with protein or vegetables with carbohydrates and not carbohydrates and proteins at the same meal. Avoid combining proteins such as beef and lobster that are popularly offered on the menus of many restaurants. Have your salad either with the meat or afterward so the hydrochloric acid can act full strength on the protein and will not convert it into stored fat due to improper digestion. Only fruits such as papaya, pineapple, apples, and grapes should be eaten with protein foods. If you are still hungry after a simple meal wait an hour or two and have another small meal. Even if you eat five or six times a day, you can avoid overeating by eating small meals and allowing plenty of time to digest food efficiently.

Nutrients

People vary in how much they want to know about nutrition. Some, addicted to evaluating food only by caloric content, have lost sight of the fact that the body needs six basic classes of nutrients to function properly. Protein, lipids (fats), carbohydrates, vitamins, minerals, and water have specific roles apart from their primary function of providing energy.

Each cell in the body contains all the nutrients needed to sustain itself; however, all cells do not require the same nutrients in identical proportion. Since cells never use more nutrients than needed, an oversupply that can't be stored or eliminated from the body within a certain time has a tendency to become toxic. If there is an insufficient amount of nutrients in the cells, on the other hand, they will stop functioning and die.

Although my nutritional regimen may sometimes be in opposition to generally accepted nutritional principles, it is common practice in bodybuilding circles. Hard training sets up stress conditions in the body, requiring strict attention to the type of foods eaten, so essential nutrients are replaced more frequently than necessary for the average person. Therefore, my approach is not based solely on theory, which can be restrictive in not recognizing body chemistry differences among people. In addition to the studies required for my PhD in nutrition and research in the field, I have paid daily attention to the effect of good nutrition on muscular growth, repair of body tissue, and power. Over a period of time this experience made me sensitive to the particular needs of my own body, so I could purposefully plan my intake of required nutrients. By using the following guidelines you should be able to do the same.

Protein

All life requires protein, the basic substance of all living cells. Most of the body's protein occurs in the form of structural units that make up muscles and connective tissues, and it forms the major part of such organs as the heart and skeletal muscles. In the average person about 30 percent of the body's supply of protein is found in the muscle tissue. With bodybuilders this figure goes up to 40–50 percent.

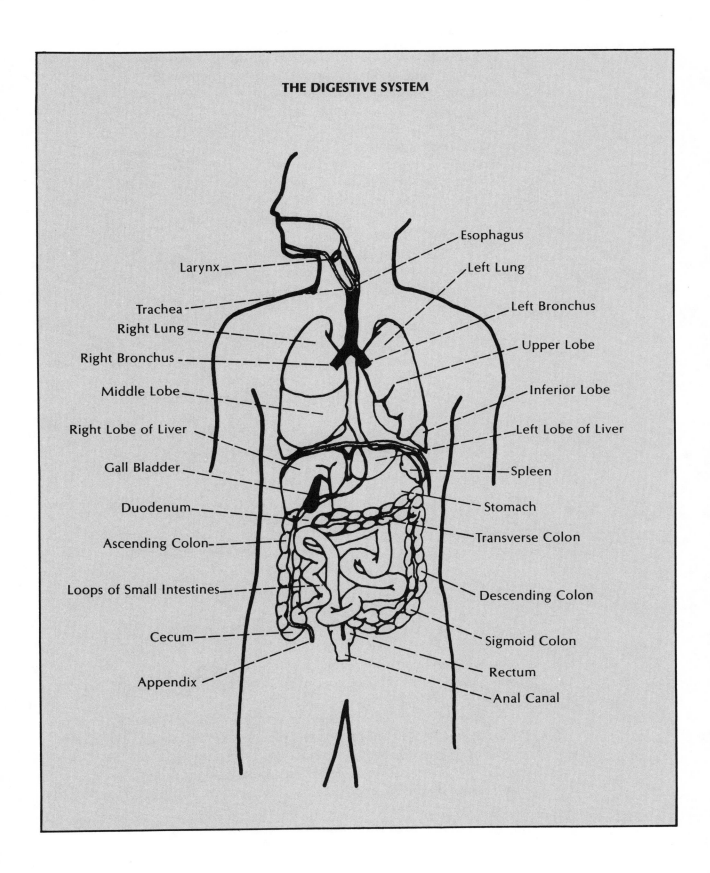

THE DIGESTIVE SYSTEM

Proteins are the best foods for building and repairing the body, with those coming from animal sources more highly efficient than those from plants. For example, you would have to eat 10 potatoes to get the same amount found in a serving of meat, since one potato yields 2 grams of protein as opposed to 20 supplied by one slice of meat or 40 in a serving of fish.

Protein is not used by the body in the form that it is eaten. Through the process of digestion it is converted into nitrogen-containing amino acids that are used by the body to make the particular kinds of proteins it needs. Of the 21 amino acids found in human protein, the body can produce only 12, which are synthesized by the glands. These are called the *nonessential amino acids* because they can be omitted if enough nitrogen and other nutrients are supplied. The essential amino acids cannot be made by the body but must be taken directly from the food we eat.

Protein is further classified as being a complete or an incomplete protein, according to its source. With the exception of soybeans, all vegetable proteins are incomplete. Being of lower biological value, they lack one or more of the essential amino acids. A complete protein is of high biological value, meaning that it comes from an animal source (fish, chicken, mammal) and contains all the essential amino acids in the right proportion needed by the body.

The quality of various proteins is measured by its digestibility, the amount and proportion of essential amino acids that are present, and its net protein utilization (NPU), which is the amount absorbed by the body. It should be noted that beef and chicken have the same absorption level with an NPU of 68 percent.

The following list will enable you to select the type of protein you should consume.

- Eggs provide the most complete protein with 88 percent of their supply absorbed by the body.
- Fish is next with an approximate 78 percent absorption level.
- Dairy products come close behind with 76 percent.
- Meat is fourth with about a 68 percent absorption level.
- Soybeans have a 48 percent absorption level.

Under normal conditions every kilogram (2.2 pounds) of body weight needs 1 gram of protein per day. If you weigh 220 pounds, a total of 100 grams is your required daily intake. Those not familiar with the composition of food may believe it is difficult to meet the recommended requirements, but it is more simple than you may realize.

For adult males the intake of protein should be 75–100 grams per day. I will give you an example of how easily this can be accomplished. The average portion of fish served in a restaurant will provide 40–50 grams of protein while a regular T-bone steak will give you 25–40. An egg contains six or seven grams, and one cup of yogurt supplies approximately eight grams. So, if you have a couple of eggs for breakfast, meat for lunch, and fish for dinner, you will have consumed about 100 grams.

Protein and Training Regimens

An extra allowance of protein is required to build muscular weight for those in heavy training. For example, a man weighing 150 pounds who trains from one to one and a half hours a day should increase his daily intake by 20–30 grams by adding one or two small protein meals to his diet program. Because of my heavy weight training, I consume huge amounts of protein daily, always careful to select the best sources. In addition to eating only prime cuts of meat, I also eat all varieties of natural cheese as well as eggs, homemade yogurt, and raw seeds and nuts.

If your consumption of protein is increased, your body does not automatically secrete more hydrochloric acid (HCl) to help digest it. Therefore, those in training who have increased their protein intake may require HCl and digestive enzyme supplements. The role of enzymes in the digestion of food is discussed later on, but bear in mind that anything can be overdone. Experiment with your body and eat what feels right to you. Certainly, you should have enough energy for training but not feel full or bloated. If you feel bloated, you may be eating too much, not digesting your food, or consuming the wrong food combinations.

Dangers of Strict Protein Diets

Those who would favor a diet restricted solely to protein should be aware they would be feeding the body but not the brain, which gets its food supply from carbohydrates and the oxygen we breathe. Unlike most other organs, the brain cannot use its store of sugar by converting it into the glucose necessary for brain functioning. It must get its sugar from the bloodstream as provided by other food elements. Lacking them, you could suffer from problems such as dizziness, slow thinking, or a high state of irritability.

In contrast, a diet limited to carbohydrates and proteins of low biological value will inhibit the body's ability to build tissue, manufacture cells, make hemoglobin, and form antibodies that fight off infection. Vegetarians risk miscombining vegetable proteins and thus failing to form complete proteins containing all the essential amino acids. After a number of years on this type of diet a person will tend to sag from the tip of the nose to the end of the ankles. This is particularly noticeable in women. The lack of complete proteins eventually causes vegetarians to lose the collagen in their connective tissues that keeps body joints smooth and flexible, and they lose the elastin, which makes repairing tissue possible. While it is possible to devise a vegetarian diet that has the nutritionally proper amino acids in balanced proportion, this demands time and knowledge.

Also to be regarded with caution are diets dependent on protein powders and tablets to supply major nutritional elements. There is a vast difference in quality between protein derived from animal sources and that from powdered concentrates and tablets. I have come to qualify the former as *live protein* and the other as *dead protein*. The key lies in the molecules of DNA found in the cells. In animal protein, even when the animal is dead, the DNA remains alive and unbroken. However, the DNA of protein powders, which originate from an animal source, are broken down during the manufacturing process. This impairs its ability to build the hundreds of different protein molecules needed for body tissue.

In addition, the digestive enzymes are inhibited by the waste products contained in these protein concentrates and do not allow them to be utilized effectively. For example, in comparing four grams of protein from an egg yolk with an equal amount of powdered protein, you will absorb about 3½ grams of protein from the egg but less than 2 from the powder. Therefore, no matter the claims made for protein powders and tablets, they should be rejected as quick and easy but ineffective substitutes for natural foods such as meat, fish, eggs, and poultry.

If, for some reason, you persist in taking protein powder, be sure to mix it with milk or water instead of fruit juices as suggested by the manufacturer. Most fruit juices contain highly concentrated sugar that does not combine with protein, causing the mixture to putrefy in the colon rather than being digested. Even sugar-free juices will ferment and turn into sugar as time goes by. A similar problem is encountered with protein tablets that are sugar-coated.

Protein Utilization

I have emphasized the digestion of protein because its efficient utilization is dependent on having all essential amino acids present at the same time and in specific proportions. Lacking even one essential amino acid causes the others, or parts of them, to become useless as they cannot be stored for future use. Instead, they break down into energy-yielding compounds and their nitrogen is excreted. As a result, the body's ability to make protein is seriously impaired.

The digestion of protein begins in the stomach with hydrochloric acid (HCl), the medium necessary for pepsin, the major stomach enzyme, to react effectively in digesting protein. The secretion of HCl does not remain constant throughout our lifetime. At the age of 65 we produce only 23 percent of the hydrochloric acid that we did at age 18. One symptom of improper protein digestion is the formation of gas. To some extent this is caused by the reduction of gastric juice, whose acid nature destroys stomach bacteria so that food can enter the intestine almost in a sterile state. Therefore, if the secretion of HCl is significantly reduced, you could have digestive problems.

I suggest taking one or two tablets of HCl to help break down protein in the stomach for proper digestion and assimilation. If you prefer, eat fruits such as papaya, pineapple, and grapes, which are rich in enzymes and effect the conversion of protein as needed for utilization.

An additional step is recommended, particularly for bodybuilders in heavy training who have increased their intake of protein. They should be certain of having enough vitamin B_6 to aid in the metabolism of protein. An increase of 250 milligrams of B_6 would be ideal to aid the conversion of protein into muscle. These should be purchased in their single form rather than as multivitamins, which contain all the B vitamins in equal proportion.

In summary, protein is needed all through life for the maintenance and repair of body tissue, to make hemoglobin, and to form the antibodies that fight infection. Significant amounts are found in meat, poultry, fish, milk, cheese, eggs, dry beans, dry peas, and nuts.

Carbohydrates

As mentioned previously, carbohydrates are the body's chief source of energy, being provided primarily by starches, sugars, and cellulose (fibrous materials). During the process of digestion some carbohydrates are converted into glucose to supply our need for immediate energy; others are stored as glycogen in the liver and muscles; the remainder are stored as adipose (fat) tissue.

Glucose, commonly called *blood sugar*, is the main product of carbohydrate digestion. Utilized mainly by the cells to furnish energy for body processes, it also supports activity and growth. Since the central nervous system is entirely dependent on glucose for energy, an adequate intake is indispensable for the functional integrity of the nerve tissue and as a source of energy for the brain.

Any glucose not immediately used by the central nervous system is carried to the liver, where it is converted into glycogen and further changed into simple sugar as required by the body. Approximately 350 grams of glycogen can be stored by the body, with one-third of the amount held in the liver and used for energy in accelerated activities of the body. The remaining two-thirds is stored mainly in the muscles and used for muscular energy.

Two or three hours of very hard training can consume the major part of the body's glycogen reserve. For this reason I stress training on alternate days when your program requires intensive workouts. In other words, if you train for two or three hours on Monday, you should not train again on Tuesday. After a heavy workout it takes about 48 hours to restore the full amount of glycogen, and you cannot train properly without it. Being aware of this, most professional athletes such as tennis players do not play the day before a competitive match so they can draw from a full supply of energy on the following day.

The role of carbohydrates in the diet has been misunderstood by many weight-conscious people who have restricted their intake out of fear of getting fat. This stems from mistaken notions regarding their nutritional value. Natural (unrefined) carbohydrates will not necessarily make you fat. For example, the highly successful Weight Watchers program features fruits and vegetables that must be consumed on a daily basis.

It is *sugar*, a form of refined carbohydrate, that really puts on the pounds. It is also sugar that makes you hungry. After eating foods such as sweet pastry, soda pop, and candy, your blood sugar level rises, and your body responds by producing a hormone called *insulin*. This hormone causes a rapid drop in your blood sugar level, which makes you hungry again within a couple of hours. Refined carbohydrates are so concentrated that they overload the system, which is equipped to store only a limited amount for energy needs. The rest is converted to fat or eliminated before becoming toxic.

In contrast, natural carbohydrates such as fresh fruits and vegetables are needed on a regular basis. A study done by the Senate Committee on Nutrition and Human Need for the United States recommended an increase in carbohydrate consumption to account for 55–60 percent of the energy (caloric) intake. As mentioned earlier, natural carbohydrates replenish energy for your nervous system, which becomes irritated without sufficient glucose to meet its needs. Therefore, it is advisable to eat fruits such as pears, apples, or grapes not only before training but also before business meetings, sports competitions, and exams, to increase your alertness and energy level. If the body lacks the store of glycogen primarily supplied by carbohydrates, it will draw energy from the protein used to build and repair body tissues. This fact should be carefully considered by those who have eliminated or severly cut back carbohydrates from their diet.

To summarize, carbohydrates furnish energy for body processes, spare proteins by supplying energy, and help the body use fats efficiently. Good sources are fruits, vegetables, whole-grain breads, and cereals. Carbohydrates obtained from fresh fruits and vegetables have greater value from the standpoint of digestibility and health.

Fats

Fat is a form of energy that is stored in the body for later use and is the primary source of muscle energy at rest—when muscles repair themselves and store energy. Everyone needs some fat to carry the fat-soluble vitamins A, D, E, and K. Fat also supplies linoleic acid, an essential fatty acid that is not manufactured by the body and is needed for the utilization of cholesterol and saturated fats.

In the process of digestion fat is split up by bile salts from the liver and gallbladder and then carried to the small intestine, where the process is completed by the enzyme lipase. Fat is stored in the body if more is absorbed than can be used immediately. The term *stored fat* does not imply that the fat eaten with a pork chop or French fries stays in one place permanently. Instead, there is a constant removal and replacement of the fatty acids in body fat. As yet, little is known concerning this constant turnover, but perhaps in time it will serve as the key to maintaining ideal weight.

One gram of fat contains nine calories, as opposed to an equal amount of protein or carbohydrate, which has four. Because fats are digested slowly, they give a pleasant feeling of fullness after being eaten, and they delay rapid development of hunger as often happens after having a meal high in refined carbohydrates. However, care should be taken to keep the total intake of fats at a moderate level because this can lead to obesity. Excessive body fat overworks the heart and vascular system and can lead to atherosclerosis.

Most hormones in the body are produced by fat cells. Female hormones are totally controlled by the amount of fat in their bodies. For example, in women the average amount of body fat should be 25 percent. If it drops below 10 percent, their bodies will stop producing the female sex hormone estrogen. In many cases women who are very thin or have a low percentage of body fat no longer produce the hormones that bring on menstruation. This condition is sometimes found among female athletes.

The amount of body fat in men ranges between 15 and 20 percent, with a large majority of men having the higher percentage. Since more women than men work at keeping their weight down, generally they are more aware of which foods contain a high percentage of fat.

Summing up, fats are a concentrated source of energy needed to carry fat-soluble vitamins. They contain more than double the number of calories of protein and carbohydrates; therefore, your daily intake of them should be kept at a low level. The most common sources are butter, margarine, oil, mayonnaise, nuts, bacon, and other fatty meats. Whole milk, eggs, chocolate, and avocados naturally contain some fat.

Cholesterol

In America I have noticed a general concern over the amount of cholesterol in the diet. Many people began regarding eggs as dangerous substances and limited their intake or entirely avoided them. It should be understood that eggs are a complete food, very rich in lecithin and choline. Lecithin helps to break down cholesterol for utilization by the body; choline promotes the metabolism of fat. If you include a reasonable number (10–20) of eggs in your weekly diet, normal levels of cholesterol are not jeopardized.

Focusing on the dark side of cholesterol has obscured its importance in hormone production and in conducting nerve impulses throughout your system. When these points are considered it becomes obvious that cholesterol should not be eliminated from your diet or other problems may result. Instead, concern should be focused on high triglyceride levels, particularly common among businessmen. Triglycerides, or the amount of fat in the blood, can cause a lack of blood flow throughout the body. The most effective way to keep their level down is to do vigorous physical exercise such as working out in a gym or running. On the other hand, a rise in their level is triggered by stress, refined sugar, and animal products such as fat.

Water

One of the most important of the six classes of nutrients is water, ranking next to air, or oxygen, in being essential for life. You can live for weeks without food, but you cannot survive without water even for a few days. Approximately three-quarters of your total body weight is made up of water, the medium for all body fluids. Being the solvent for all products of digestion, it holds them in solution so they can pass through the intestinal wall into the bloodstream for use thoughout the body.

If you become dehydrated, the cells also become dehydrated, impairing their ability to build tissue and utilize energy efficiently. Without enough water, toxic products build up in the bloodstream, you don't sweat, and blood volume decreases so you transport less oxygen and nutrients through your body. This results in your muscles becoming weak and feeling tired.

Almost everyone drinks less water than is required. Eight to 10 glasses are recommended for the average person, but when exercising you need far more fluids. When you consume extra vitamins, protein, or alcohol, more water is required.

Supplements

Most people believe a well-balanced diet eliminates the need for taking extra vitamins and minerals. Yet during recent years the soil in this country, and in most of the world, has become devitalized so most food grown is depleted of minerals. In my opinion, it is very important to supplement your diet with vitamins and minerals, having minerals rank first in importance because they are the building blocks of the body and essential to proper absorption and utilization of vitamins.

Because there is a good deal of competition in selling and advertising nutritional supplements, I have set forth a few guidelines to help in your selection:

1. Check the date of expiration stamped on most bottles of supplements, choosing only those dated two or more years ahead of the purchase date. Ordinarily, manufacturers make a supply that, according to them, should be good for three years. In other words, if their product is made in 1982, they state its viable condition will last until 1985. However, if you are purchasing supplements in 1982, do not buy any with expiration dates in 1983; those marked 1984 or 1985 have more stable nutritional value.

2. Buy high-potency products. This will eliminate the need for taking several tablets or capsules daily, so you will get less of the coating and binder.

3. Read the label, choosing only those supplements identified as free from additives such as artificial color, preservatives, and sugar. If this is not specified, most likely additives were used to give the supplements eye appeal or to make them more palatable.

Some consideration should be given to the problem of stress as it relates to the glandular system. When people are under stress from overwork, anxiety, improper nutrition, or inadequate sleep, their endocrine glands may become exhausted. Composed of eight differ-ent glands (pituitary, thyroid, parathyroid, pancreas, adrenal, ova-ries, testes, and pineal) the endocrines work in harmony with the nervous system to control and coordinate all body activities. If the endocrine system, which secretes hormones, is out of balance, your body chemistry is also upset.

Whatever the type of stress, the body immediately tries to repair any damage done to the system, but it cannot do so unless all nu-trients are supplied. After checking with your doctor, take glandular supplements to feed the glands and reactivate them. Supplements are available for either individual glands or all of them collectively. Helping to rehabilitate the glands will make them more resistant to stress. For example, glandular supplements may be needed by men who work very hard, possibly straining or overworking their adre-nals, which are essential to life. Some "workaholics" have damaged their adrenals by maintaining an unreasonable pace, through poor nutrition, and through lack of sleep. Others, who are very active, may have hyperthyroidism, overactivity of the thyroid gland.

Before buying any supplements, have a complete blood study and hair mineral analysis done to determine your needs. The results should be interpreted by a professional so a food supplement pro-gram can be designed to correct deficiencies. The table on page 111 will provide guidelines for the average person not under a great deal of stress. When you are anxiety-ridden for prolonged periods of time your nutrient requirements are higher because the body uses them rapidly. Negative emotions such as fear, fatigue, anger, and obses-sive worry also inhibit the normal secretion of enzymes and hor-mones. Therefore, you should relax before eating if emotionally disrupted or your system will be unable to utilize the full nutritional value of your meal.

General Food Program

Many individuals excuse themselves from adhering to a sound nutri-tional program on the grounds that it takes too much time or effort. Yet in most cases it is far easier to prepare food high in nutritional value than to take a frozen block of something from the freezer and have it ready in time for dinner. For instance, it takes approximately one or two minutes to steam fresh spinach, but 10–14 minutes to thaw and cook the frozen variety. A baked potato requires only the effort of placing it in the oven with no pots or pans to wash, while the preparation of mashed potatoes demands having them peeled, sliced, and mixed with other ingredients. It is far easier to slice an orange into four quarters and simply eat it than to mix a can of frozen

Suggested Daily Intake of Vitamins and Minerals

Vitamin A	25,000 IU	Phosphorus	150 mg
Vitamin D	400 IU	Iron	20 mg
Vitamin C	1,000 mg	Iodine	20 mg
Vitamin E	1,000 IU	Copper	2 mg
Vitamin B$_1$	100 mg	Zinc	25 mg
Vitamin B$_2$	100 mg	Manganese	20 mg
Vitamin B$_6$	150 mg	Chromium	750 mcg
Vitamin B$_{12}$	300 mcg	Selenium	100 mcg
Niacin or niacinamide	100 mg	Beatine HCl	100 mg
Pantothenic acid	100 mg	Pepsin	50 mg
Para-aminobenzoic acid	75 mg	Bromelain	50 mg
Choline	100 mg	Ox bile	30 mg
Inositol	100 mg	Pancreas substance	100 mg
Folic acid	400 mcg	Papain	50 mg
Biotin	100 mcg	Protease	100 mg
Calcium	1,000 mg	Amylase	25 mg
Magnesium	500 mg	Lipase	25 mg
Potassium	200 mg		

concentrate with three cans of water and stir until well blended. Broiling or baking chicken takes far less time and effort than dipping pieces in flour and breadcrumbs before frying, and fixing a salad with fresh vegetables and tuna for protein takes about three hours less than preparing and simmering a pot of beef stew.

In shopping for appropriate foods, extra time may be required to read labels on bread, cereals, grains, and other foods to select those containing little or no additives, but once you are familiar with the brand, no additional effort is required.

Foods to Eat

Listed below are my recommendations for a general food program of high nutritional value, along with guidelines for selection and preparation of various items.

Beverages

Drink mineral water, beer, white or red wine, champagne, a limited amount of coffee and tea. You should try to drink a total of 8–10 glasses of water daily (carbonated beverages do not count).

Fruit and Fruit Juices

Eat fresh fruit once or twice daily with one choice being a citrus fruit. Because whole fruit adds bulk to the diet, it is better than fruit juice. If the juice is freshly made, however, it may be substituted for one serving of fruit. Dried fruit has a high sugar and calorie content; therefore, those wanting to lose weight should avoid it.

Vegetables

One or more servings of fresh, raw vegetables should be eaten daily and lightly steamed vegetables once, with an occasional baked potato. I have a large raw vegetable salad twice a day. Guard against overcooking vegetables since this robs them of their unique flavor and nutritional value. Fruit and vegetables are rich in minerals and vitamins, providing an excellent source of bulk when eaten raw.

Eggs

Have at least one egg a day. Eggs are the best source of protein and are highly versatile for combining with different foods.

Poultry

Buy poultry that is fresh rather than frozen and try to find a market that sells poultry raised without hormones or other injections. Many health food stores now carry it. Before cooking, remove the skin because of its high fat content. To retain the high nutritional value, either bake or broil poultry with vegetable seasonings. It is a great source of protein and is low in fat.

Meat

Eat only lean cuts of beef, lamb, and veal, trimming off all fat before cooking. When having meat in a restaurant, be sure to cut off all the fat before eating it.

Seafood

Fish is the next best source of protein after eggs. It is generally low in fats, high in protein and amino acids. Seafood is particularly high in trace minerals. When you eat canned fish, be sure it is packed in water, not oil.

Oils and Fats

In the United States our consumption of fats makes up more than 50 percent of our daily diet. Butter contributes to this high percentage and should be avoided as much as possible. The normal daily consumption should be about 30 percent, but should not drop below 10 percent. Try to eliminate all fried foods, mayonnaise, margarine, and almost all oils and oil dressings. I make an exception, using a small amount of pure olive oil and vinegar as a salad dressing.

Bread

Whole wheat, stoneground, pita, and seven-grain are the breads I recommend. Here it is important to read the label and select brands containing no sugar or other additives.

Cereal

Seven-grain granola cereals are an excellent source of minerals and B-complex vitamins. Those trying to lose weight should eat cereal only two or three times per week.

Grains

Eat natural brown rice, raw bran flakes, and other natural whole grains that are not processed or refined.

Dairy Products

Most dairy products are not properly digested by persons over 10 years of age. In my opinion all dairy products should be avoided; however, a small amount may be good for nourishing intestinal flora, the bacteria that regulate and combat bacteria disruptive to the intestine.

Raw Seeds and Nuts

Since nuts and seeds are high in calories, they should not be eaten in excess if you are trying to lose weight. They do, however, supply essential fatty acids and are high in some trace minerals and B-complex vitamins.

Foods to Avoid

Food preservatives such as nitrates and nitrites, white flour, artificial coloring and flavoring, sugar, and hydrogenated fat should be avoided. It may be difficult to eliminate many of these from your diet totally, but by carefully reading labels you can sharply reduce the amount ingested. Of all of them, sugar is the most potentially damaging item, causing problems that range from hypoglycemia to hormone disorders.

Eating Out

When dining in a restaurant, always try to order simple foods that are not adorned with sauces or fried with a coating of batter or breadcrumbs. This is usually easier when you know the specialties of area restaurants in advance, so you can avoid any not serving simple food. I always prefer to order fish, but good fish is not easily found in a majority of restaurants, so I order meat either broiled or plain roasted, a salad with oil and vinegar dressing, and a baked potato or steamed rice. I do not choose items from the menu by virtue of their grandiose descriptions but by their volume of protein. The best choices, in order, are fish, eggs, and meat.

The easiest way to avoid the temptation of sauce-laden foods, platters of garlic bread, hot fudge sundaes, and pies topped with whipped cream is to decide exactly what to order before entering the restaurant. A mind firmly fixed in one direction is less liable to be swayed by an enticing list of menu items. Also, if it does not offend any ravenously hungry dinner companions, ask the waiter to remove the basket of bread and butter from the table. Have the dressing or any condiments served as side dishes to avoid having your food drenched in them by overly liberal cooks or kitchen aides. And, as mentioned earlier, try to relax before eating so your appetite is directed by actual hunger rather than emotions.

Life Extension

Staying young and extending your life span is certainly a major goal. In recent years a great deal of research on life extension has been conducted on both animals and humans in many industrialized countries. The results show that humans are biologically capable of living from 120 to 150 years. Yet too many lives are shortened because daily mistakes become cumulative over a number of years. Smoking and certain beverages, like diet sodas and hard alcohol, rob their users of precious life each day.

The prime factors inhibiting life extension are the quantity and quality of foods we eat. In tests conducted with animals physiologically similar to humans, it was found that their life expectancy doubled when their food ration was cut by two-thirds. Here in America the greatest danger of a shortened life span comes from overeating, especially foods with no nutritional value. Therefore, bear in mind that your life extension depends on eating less food and being certain it is of high quality and contains the essential amino acids, vitamins, and minerals.

Vitamins

Unlike carbohydrates, fats, and proteins, vitamins are not needed in bulk to build muscle or tissue. They are, however, essential for proper growth and maintenance of health. Like hormones, they regulate the body processes. As in the case of trace minerals (iodine, for example), the presence or absence of vitamins in small amounts can prove the difference between good and bad health.

Plants manufacture their own vitamins. Animals obtain theirs from plants or other animals that eat plants; a few manufacture some of the vitamins they need. This is not the case with human beings, who must depend on minute quantities existent in all natural foods. As contrasted with carbohydrates, fats, and proteins, which are broken down into other substances, vitamins retain their original form in the body. They serve an important role in the machinery of all cells to bring about certain changes and processes. For instance, vitamin B in itself is not fattening like large amounts of carbohydrates and fatty foods. But a very thin person suffering from digestive problems might gain weight, having vitamin B in the digestive tract to regulate the metabolic process and utilization of food.

Vitamins are divided into two groups based on their solubility. The fat-soluble vitamins (A, D, E, and K) are found in foods containing a high percentage of lipids (fats). The water-soluble vitamins (B-complex and C) cannot be stored by the body and require constant replenishment.

Minerals

As previously mentioned, minerals are the building blocks of the body. They are also needed for overall mental and physical functioning, feeding the nerves in order to make you tranquil, strong, and vibrant. Theirs is the power to control body liquids and to permit other nutrients to pass into the bloodstream. By drawing substances in and out of the cells, they aid in keeping blood and tissue from becoming either too acid or too alkaline.

Minerals are as important to us as vitamins. Yet their value is often overlooked, neglected, or underestimated. To assure more complete assimilation of minerals by the body, try to get chelated minerals, which are 10 times more digestible than nonchelated.

Note: The symptoms noted on the vitamin and mineral table that follows can occur only when the daily intake of these nutrients falls below the minimum daily requirement over a long period of time. These nonspecific symptoms alone are not proof of nutritional deficiencies but may be caused by any great number of conditions or may have functional causes. If the symptoms persist, they may indicate a condition other than a vitamin or mineral deficiency. If any of these symptoms persist, it would be wise to consult your physician.

VITAMINS AND MINERALS
VITAMINS

Vitamin	Best Natural Sources	Functions	Deficiency Symptoms	Adversely Affects Nutrient
Vitamin A	Fish, liver, oil, eggs, dairy products	Builds resistance to infection, especially respiratory tract. Promotes growth and vitality. Helps maintain healthy skin and outer layers of tissues and organs. Essential for strong eyesight and night vision.	Night blindness, susceptibility to infections, lack of appetite and vigor	Alcohol, caffeine, mineral oil, excessive iron, vitamin D deficiency
Vitamin B₁	Organ meats, eggs, yeast, green leafy vegetables, whole-grain cereals	Promotes growth and digestion. Essential for normal functioning of nerve tissues, muscles, heart. Aids in metabolism of carbohydrates and fats. Helps maintain healthy nervous system.	Loss of appetite, weakness, nervous irritability, mental depression, weight loss, insomnia	Tobacco, alcohol, caffeine, stress, fever

Vitamin	Best Natural Sources	Functions	Deficiency Symptoms	Adversely Affects Nutrient
Vitamin B₂	Milk, liver, fish, eggs, yeast, some green vegetables	Essential for healthy eyes, skin, mouth. Helps metabolize proteins, fats, and carbohydrates. Necessary for blood and antibody formation.	Itching and burning eyes, cracking at corners of lips, bloodshot eyes	Sugar, alcohol, caffeine, tobacco
Vitamin B₆	Eggs, beef, organ meats, brewer's yeast, bran, wheat germ	Ensures proper synthesis of amino acids. Aids metabolism of protein and fats. Prevents nausea. A natural diuretic.	Nervousness, insomnia, skin eruptions, irritability, depression	Tobacco, caffeine, alcohol, birth control pills, radiation
Pantothenic Acid	Organ meats, whole grains, green vegetables	Improves body's ability to withstand hard training. Prevents fatigue. Helps build body cells, maintain normal skin tone, utilize vitamins.	Skin abnormalities, dizzy spells, digestive disturbances	Sugar, alcohol, caffeine
Folic Acid	Vegetables, egg yolks, wheat germ, organ meats	Stimulates production of HCl. Aids in protein metabolism. Essential to formation of red blood cells through action on blood marrow	Nutritional anemia, reproductive disorders, graying and loss of hair	Stress, tobacco, alcohol, caffeine
Choline	Egg yolks, yeast, liver, wheat germ, beef heart, green vegetables	Minimizes excess fat deposits in liver. Aids in fat metabolism, normal nerve transmission. Maintains health of hair and thymus glands.	Cirrhosis, fatty degeneration of liver, high blood pressure	Alcohol, sugar, caffeine

Vitamin	Best Natural Sources	Functions	Deficiency Symptoms	Adversely Affects Nutrient
Inositol	Liver, brewer's yeast, citrus fruits, wheat germ	Performs functions similar to choline. Helpful in brain cell nutrition. Lowers cholesterol levels in the blood. Prevents thinning hair and baldness.	High cholesterol, constipation, skin problems	Alcohol, sugar, corn, caffeine, antibiotics
Biotin	Liver, beef heart, eggs, cheese, milk, beef	Related to metabolism of fat and conversion of certain amino acids. Good for healthy skin, hair, muscles.	Extreme exhaustion, drowsiness, muscle pains, loss of appetite	Caffeine, alcohol, raw egg whites
Niacin	Liver, lean meat, whole wheat, milk, nuts	Aids in functioning of nervous system, metabolism of carbohydrates, normal function of gastrointestinal tract. Dilates blood vessels.	Pellagra, headaches, depression, nervous system dysfunction	Caffeine, sugar, alcohol, antibiotics, corn
Vitamin B$_{12}$	Liver, eggs, cheese, milk, beef, kidneys	Helps formation and regeneration of red blood cells. Essential in metabolizing protein, fat, and carbohydrates.	Fatigue, nutritional anemia, poor appetite	Most laxatives, tobacco, alcohol, caffeine
Vitamin B$_{15}$	Grains, pumpkin and sesame seeds, brown rice, brewer's yeast	Used by Russian athletes for increased energy. Promotes protein metabolism, particularly in heart muscles. Regulates metabolism of fat and sugar.	Fatigue, hypoglycemia, dizziness, possibly retarded growth	Caffeine, alcohol sugar

Vitamin	Best Natural Sources	Functions	Deficiency Symptoms	Adversely Affects Nutrient
Vitamin B₁₇ (laetrile)	Whole kernels of apricots, plums, nectarines, cherries, peaches, apples	Popular in Europe. Claims have been made that it has cancer-controlling properties.	Unknown	Unknown
Vitamin C	Citrus fruits berries, tomatoes	Necessary for healthy teeth, gums, bones. Promotes wound healing. Strengthens connective tissue. Aids free movement when exercising, because body warms up faster, and thins out synovial fluids lubricating the joints.	Soft gums, tooth decay, loss of appetite, muscular weakness, anemia	Tobacco, sugar, stress, aspirin, antibiotics
Vitamin D	Dairy products, fish, fish liver oil	Regulates use of calcium and phosphorus; therefore, necessary for proper formation of teeth and bones. Best utilized if taken with vitamin A. Maintains stable nervous system.	Tooth decay, rickets, lack of vigor, muscular weakness.	Mineral oil
Vitamin E	Eggs, wheat germ, vegetable oils, leafy greens, whole wheat	Essential role in oxygenating the tissues. Reduces need for oxygen. Dilates blood vessels. Prevents formation of excessive scar tissue.	Degeneration of sex hormones, dry and dull hair, sterility	Rancid fat and oil, mineral oil

MINERALS

Mineral	Best Natural Sources	Functions	Deficiency Symptoms	Adversely Affects Nutrient
Calcium	Dairy products, fish, chicken, meat, whole grains, shellfish, liver	Aids muscle growth and contraction, nerve transmission. Builds and maintains bones and teeth. Tranquilizes nerves; aids vitality and endurance. Relaxes cramps from hard training. Extra 1,000 mg needed for every hour of training.	Appetite and weight loss, stunted growth, rickets, nervous disorders, mental sluggishness, fatigue	Lack of exercise, stress, lack of HCl, lack of magnesium, white sugar foods
Phosphorus	All natural foods	Present in every cell, plays role in almost every chemical reaction in body. Aids growth of bones and teeth, growth and repair of cells, synthesis of protein, carbohydrate, fat.	Loss of weight and appetite, nervous disorders, general fatigue, poor formation of bones and teeth	White sugar foods, excessive aluminum, magnesium, and iron
Copper	Seafood, beans, mushrooms, nuts, raisins	Aids manufacture of hemoglobin. Carries oxygen in blood. Present in body-building enzymes. Aids body healing and bone formation.	Anemia, weakness, hair loss, poor respiration	Excessive zinc
Magnesium	Fruits, nuts, seeds	Along with calcium, is vital for athletes in prevention of muscle cramps. Regulates blood sugar levels. Aids function of nerves and muscles.	Nervous irritability, tremors, depression	Unknown

Mineral	Best Natural Sources	Functions	Deficiency Symptoms	Adversely Affects Nutrient
Sulphur	Fish, eggs, beef, beans, cabbage, Brussels sprouts	Works with B-complex vitamins needed for strong nerve health. Promotes good skin, hair, and nails. Causes liver to secrete bile.	Unknown	Unknown
Manganese	Egg yolks, nuts, green leafy vegetables	Works with other minerals to create normal bone structure. Aids digestion and utilization of food, muscular reflexes, sex hormone production.	Dizziness, sterility, stunted growth, male impotence	Excessive phosphorus and calcium
Sodium	Table salt	Renders other blood minerals more soluble, preventing their being clogged or deposited in blood distribution system. Provides strength to muscles so they can contract.	Stomach and intestinal gas, weight loss, muscle shrinkage	Unknown
Potassium	Potatoes, bananas, vegetables, seeds	Joins with phosphorus in sending oxygen to brain. Works with sodium in normalizing heartbeat and feeding muscular system. Necessary for normal muscle tone, heart action, and enzyme reaction.	Weakness, nervous disorders, insomnia, tendency toward muscle damage	Most diuretics, sugar, caffeine, alcohol, most laxatives

Mineral	Best Natural Sources	Functions	Deficiency Symptoms	Adversely Affects Nutrient
Chlorine	Table salt	Keeps joints and tendons youthful by helping distribution of hormones. Cleans toxic waste from system. Stimulates production of HCl.	Poor muscular contractibility, hair and tooth loss, faulty digestion	Unknown
Iodine	Seafood, vegetables, kelp	Regulates body's production of energy. Aids proper functioning of thyroid gland. Stimulates rate of metabolism, helping body burn off excess fat.	Goiter, obesity, sluggish metabolism, lowered mentality	Unknown
Zinc	Meat, eggs	Important to body-building because little is found in natural foods due to soil depletion. Needed for absorption of vitamins, especially B-complex. Produces energy. Governs controllability in muscles.	Hair loss, enlarged prostate, poor wound healing	Excessive calcium, alcohol

Six

Sports Training Programs

Obviously the best way to improve in any sport is to master the technique and skills required and continue to play regularly. Whatever your game, the programs that follow will give you muscularity along with the agility required for most sports. Building stamina by weight training will give you the endurance and power needed for a dynamic performance. Your increased strength will improve coordination, balance, reaction time, and the ability to change direction rapidly while moving fast.

Each of the training programs in this chapter is geared directly toward improving a particular sport, since each one causes certain muscles to be overused while others are not used at all. This often creates a muscular imbalance, and the athlete should correct it by training with weights. Therefore, a high number of repetitions are given for certain exercises to bring opposing pairs of muscles into balance. To achieve the maximum results the exercises should be done in the order given.

In general, light weights are used to facilitate doing the high number of repetitions. If you need to pause more than 30–45 seconds between sets, it probably means the weights are too heavy, so scale down the poundage a little until the whole program can be finished without stopping.

Although you can work out before playing your particular sport, it is better to play first and train afterward. Allow yourself at least one day of rest between workouts and go through the routine three times a week. All the programs can be followed unchanged for six months. By then, assuming you've kept up with your original sport, you're going to start looking for tougher competition.

Arm Wrestling

While arm wrestling appears to be a test of sheer man-to-man strength, a good deal of skill and acquired proficiency are needed to win. A competitor who trains his muscles is capable of defeating opponents who are bigger and stronger than himself. Abraham Lincoln, who was very thin and lanky, had a reputation of being very good at it. This routine will toughen up the muscles and ligaments of the forearms and wrists for the particular stresses occurring in arm wrestling.

Bench Press	3 × 10
Cross Flye	3 × 10
Pulldown	3 × 15
Bent-Over Lateral Raise	3 × 10
Lateral Raise	3 × 10
Triceps Pushdown	3 × 10
Forearm Exercise	5 × 20

Backpacking

Unlike other sports, in which you expend great efforts for several hours and then head for the showers, backpacking places demand on your stamina from sunrise to sunset. Even when a long day of trekking uphill and downhill with a heavy pack is over, there still remains the work of setting up camp, cooking dinner, and washing up before stretching out on the hard ground for a night's sleep. Of course, the joy of traveling over territory not everyone treads far outweighs the physical demands of this rugged sport.

Weightlifting will build the muscle endurance and stamina needed to keep going without undue fatigue, especially on rough trails when making your way through brush and scrambling up steep banks. This routine will work your legs, arms, shoulders, back—everything that needs strengthening for hiking endurance.

Squat	3 × 50
Leg Extension	3 × 25
Pulldown	3 × 20
Triceps Pulldown	3 × 15
Forearm	3 × 25
Sit-Up	3 × 20
Leg Raise	3 × 20
Lying Side Leg Raise	3 × 20
Side Bend	3 × 20

Baseball

Since baseball is a game in which inches count, you need to perform exercises that improve your speed of movement. Your throwing ability can be developed to some degree through weight training exercises. More importantly, the proper routine can be helpful in preventing and correcting the muscular imbalances that are common among baseball players since they use one side of the body more than the other, particularly while pitching.

If you are a pitcher or an outfielder, the shoulder and triceps exercises in the routine will be helpful, provided you continue throwing the ball as usual. Weight training will be most helpful for batters because their muscles need the type of training that puts the snap and rotation moves into a smooth, level swing.

Cross Flye	2 × 15
Bent-Over Lateral Raise	3 × 15
Lateral Raise	3 × 15
Triceps Pushdown	3 × 15
Wrist Curl	3 × 15
Leg Extension	3 × 15
Calf Raise	3 × 25
Sit-Up	3 × 25
Leg Raise	3 × 25
Leg Stretching	2 × 20
Side Bend	2 × 20
Speed Running	2–3 miles

Basketball

At one time basketball players believed the myth about bodybuilding making men muscle-bound and kept away from weight training because their sport emphasized quickness. They eventually came to discover, however, that the muscle strength and endurance needed for this fast-paced game could be developed most quickly by training with weights. Now regular routines have been developed for teams playing at the high school, college, and pro levels.

Most basketball players have long muscles that need to be strengthened through weight training. Certainly they will profit by increasing their leaping ability and stamina. Those whose rebounding abilities are vital to their teams can train successfully to build gripping power and gain muscular weight to throw around under the boards. The smaller players have used weight training to develop their aggressiveness, speed, and agility.

Although you can work out before or after basketball training, it is best not to exercise before competing.

Hamstring Stretch	1 × 25
Calf Stretch	1 × 25
Side Bend	1 × 25
Triceps Pushdown	4 × 15
Incline Bench Press	3 × 25
Pulldown	3 × 15
Bent-Over Lateral Raise	3 × 15
Leg Extension	3 × 20
Calf Raise	4 × 20
Jump Squat	2 × 10
Sit-Up	3 × 25
Leg Raise	3 × 25

Jump Rope—Up to 10 minutes. This is still one of the greatest exercises for legs, footwork, agility, hand/eye coordination, stamina, and wind.

Speed Running—Up to 2 miles. For basketball running 2 miles is much better than jogging 4.

Bowling

This popular sport was inherited from Germany about 350 AD. The original bowling pin was a war club carried everywhere by peasants. Even into church. Priests, trying to make the idea of Satan real, developed a ritual where each peasant stood his war club in a corner and tried to knock it down with a large block or ball. Since the club represented the devil, peasants were considered virtuous if they knocked it down, but sinful if they left it standing.

Fortunately for many bowlers, no consideration is given to this ritual today—however, the game still demands accuracy and control. A good delivery form is based on a good sense of balance that can maintain a smooth, pendulum swing while avoiding sidewheeling. Loss of balance most often contributes to the foot sticking before reaching, rather than sliding to, the foul line.

Bowling form causes certain muscles to be exercised more than others. Some muscles tighten from the stress of shifting your weight almost entirely to the front foot. Because a good performance requires all parts of the body to function well, this program was designed to balance your muscles equally and to increase stamina.

Leg Extension	3 × 20
Pulldown	3 × 20
Bent-Over Lateral Raise	3 × 10
Lateral Raise	3 × 10
Triceps Pushdown	3 × 15
Wrist Curl	3 × 15
Standing Side Bend	2 × 40
Back stretch for one minute	

Boxing and Karate

I began my athletic careet as a boxer. Wanting to increase my strength and endurance for a better performance in the ring, I started working with weights. Every day I shadow-boxed a couple of rounds, holding a 2½-pound dumbbell in each hand to strengthen my punch and to increase my ability to carry my fists high through a long bout. My performance so improved that I won my last 19 fights with a first- or second-round knockout, which led me to the title of lightweight boxing champion of Italy.

Although the blows in karate are delivered with the feet as well as the hands and to different target areas, you will use about the same footwork, moves, and muscles as a boxer. The power and stamina needed for both sports can be developed using this workout routine.

Seated Leg Stretching	2 × 25
Side Bend	2 × 25
Bent-Over Lateral Raise	2 × 25
Triceps Pushdown	4 × 25
Leg Extension	3 × 25
Calf Raise	3 × 25
Calf Stretching	2 × 10
Hamstring Stretching	2 × 10
Weight Boxing—3 3-minute rounds, with 2 5-pound dumbbells or plates	
Jumping Rope—3–5 3-minute rounds	

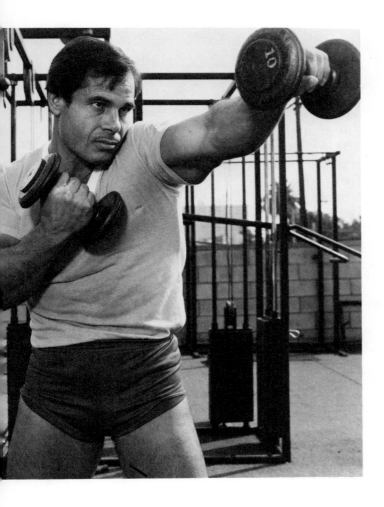

Dancing

Dancing is one of the best activities for keeping the entire body coordinated and flexible. The rhythmic, flowing movement is also beneficial for the joint/ligament structures. In addition, a session of energetic dancing can burn off from 300–400 calories, and improve cardiovascular efficiency if done on a regular basis. The underlying principle of aerobic routines incorporates swing, folk, rock, and ballet steps.

Like any sport, dancing is most enjoyable when you are in top shape and can enjoy the pure pleasure of body movement without huffing and puffing to keep up with your partner. This program will strengthen and balance the entire body. Particular attention is given to stretching exercises for developing muscular flexibility and suppleness.

Pulldown	3 × 15
Bent-Over Lateral Raise	3 × 10
Lateral Raise	3 × 10
Triceps Pushdown	3 × 15
Leg Extension	3 × 20
Calf Raise	3 × 20
Back Leg Stretch	1 minute each leg
Calf Stretch	1 minute each leg
Seated Stretch	1 minute each leg
Running	2 miles, 3 times a week

Football

Essential to the running game of the offense are the skills of a running back; therefore, he should do a wide variety of leg exercises to develop the speed, agility, and balance needed to start quickly and to change directions in an instant. Because he is the target of some of the hardest tackles in football, a running back should also have a powerful body to withstand the defense as it hits hard to stop him from going those extra yards.

Linebackers must be big enough to fight off blockers, yet fast enough to get to the ball carrier or to defend against passes. Since linebackers and linemen both need more power, I suggest placing greater emphasis on Squats, Bench Presses, and Deadlifts because these are powerlifting exercises.

Whatever your position on the team, you should determine your own needs within the program to improve your performance on the field. These exercises are targeted specifically for football players, and I suggest emphasizing those that will best serve in meeting your personal goals.

Hamstring Stretch	1 × 20
Side Bend	1 × 20
Calf Stretch	1 × 20
Squat	3 × 15

It is important to do the full squat. Here you can't use maximum weight as for the bent-leg version.

Front Squat	3 × 15
Straight-Leg Deadlift	3 × 10
Leg Extension	4 × 25

This is the best exercise to strengthen and protect the knees.

Leg Curl	2 × 25
Bench Press	3 × 15
Incline Bench Press	2 × 15
Barbell Rowing	3 × 15
Pulldown	3 × 15
Pullover	2 × 15

This is an excellent exercise for the rib cage.

Bent-Over Lateral Raise	4 × 10
Lateral Raise	4 × 10
Triceps Pushdown	5 × 10
Wrist Curl	2 × 15
Sit-Up	4 × 25
Leg Raise	4 × 25

Repeat the stretching exercises.

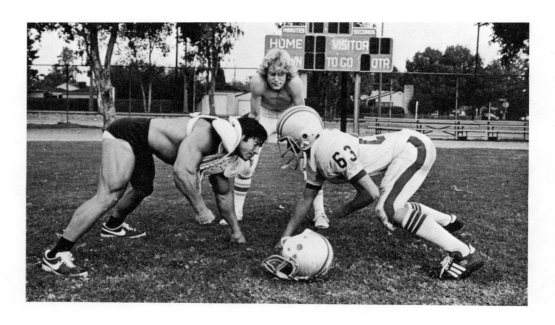

Golf

Golf places little stress on the heart and lungs. For this reason many men who were active in other sports switch to golf in later life. Some may feel they no longer need the level of physical fitness required in more vigorous sports such as tennis, skiing, and basketball. However, every golfer wants to play a super game, and this requires good conditioning. Every golfer should have good trunk strength, flexibility, endurance, and a certain amount of power. Your grip should be firm enough to withstand a high-speed swing without losing its discipline over the club, since the strength of the grip establishes the entire power of the swing.

By adhering to this program you will condition your upper body, strengthen your grip, and help prevent tennis elbow, which is the bane of many golfers as well as tennis players. The exercises for your back should be helpful in preventing backaches if you depart too far from a simple and natural swing.

Lunge	3 × 20
Pulldown	3 × 20
Bent-Over Lateral Raise	3 × 10
Lateral Raise	3 × 10
Triceps Pushdown	3 × 15
Side Bend	2 × 25
Back Leg Stretch	1 × 10

Hockey

Hockey requires stamina. Called "the fastest game on two feet," it requires players to skate up to 30 miles an hour when in full stride. The puck, after a hard slap shot by a hockey superstar, has been timed at 120 miles an hour. Unlike other sports, there are no time-outs or rest periods until the referee blows the whistle.

These exercises are excellent for building the stamina and muscle endurance needed for this fast-paced sport and to withstand the physical contact from body checks. The routine places emphasis on conditioning the legs for hard, fast skating and making quick starts and stops. The arm exercises are geared toward developing strength in handling and controlling the stick.

Squat	3 × 25
Leg Press	3 × 20
Leg Extension	4 × 25
Leg Curl	2 × 25
Calf Raise	4 × 20
Front Calf Raise	4 × 20
Wrist Curl	4 × 20
Barbell Rowing	3 × 15
Lateral Raise	3 × 15
Leg Stretching	2 × 20
Side Bend	2 × 20
Sit-Up	2 × 20

Running

This routine will work the upper part of your body first to get extra blood up there as early as possible. Once you actually begin running, the blood will go to your legs.

Although your legs will be doing all the work, it is necessary to train your upper body for the following reasons: (1) your legs will become even more disproportionately strong than they are without these exercises; (2) development of your upper body will help in resisting the tension that occurs naturally in running; and (3) developing powerful arm thrust will actually help you stride better.

Bench Press	3 × 20
Barbell Rowing	2 × 20
Pulldown	2 × 20
Bent-Over Lateral Raise	3 × 10
Lateral Raise	3 × 10
Triceps Pushdown	4 × 10
Dumbbell Curl	2 × 10
Forearm Curl	2 × 15
Leg Extension	4 × 50
Lunge	4 × 40
Squat	2 × 25
Calf Raise	5 × 40
Front Calf Raise	5 × 40

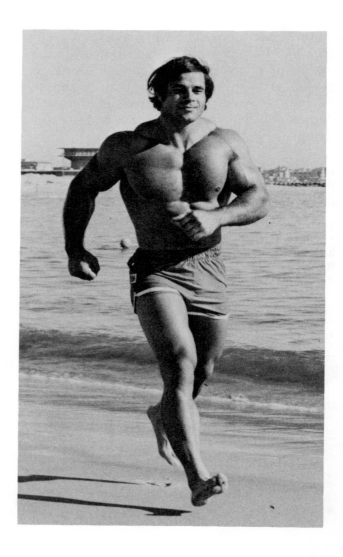

Skiing

Most skiers can go to the slopes only infrequently; therefore, it is important that they exercise regularly to ward off stiffness and prevent injuries. *Endurance* and *stamina* are key words when it comes to skiing because they postpone the onset of fatigue. You can be in trouble if the quadriceps muscles at the top of the thigh become tired and you straighten your knees to rest them.

This routine places emphasis on strengthening the leg muscles to help in edge control, unweighting, mogul hopping, and staying forward on your skis. The Calf Raises are a great Achilles tendon stretcher and develop flexibility of the ankle joints. Equally important are exercises for conditioning the upper body. Strength is needed in the arms, shoulders, and back for pole plants, climbing on skis, initiating turns, and particularly for double poling when cross-country skiing. By working out regularly you will achieve the efficient functioning of all systems in the body necessary for a dynamic sense of balance.

Lunge	3 × 25
Squat	4 × 25
Leg Extension	4 × 25
Leg Curl	1 × 25
Calf Raise	4 × 25
Front Calf Raise	4 × 25
Bench Press	3 × 20
Pulldown	3 × 20
Chins in Front of Neck	3 × 10
Lateral Raise	3 × 10
Triceps Pushdown	3 × 10
Wrist Curl	3 × 10
Abdominal Training—the next 3 exercises are done in rotation.	
Sit-Up	4 × 25
Leg Raise	4 × 25
Side Bend	4 × 25
Stretching—the next 2 exercises are done in rotation.	
Leg Stretch	2 × 25
Calf Stretch	2 × 25

Soccer

Fundamentally, soccer is a game of speed and ball control. In addition to team practice, most professionals work out alone several hours a day to improve their skills and build the endurance needed for playing this fast-paced game. The difference between mere performance and total involvement depends on the ability to draw on reserves of energy when it seems impossible to go another step. By training as fast as possible you will build the endurance and stamina needed to play 90 minutes without tiring significantly.

Since the most important movement is speeding off the mark, emphasis is placed here on exercises for the legs. The stretching exercises will help in lengthening your stride so fewer steps are needed to cover the same ground. Also included are three exercises for the triceps and shoulders for developing the gripping and throwing strength of goaltenders.

Leg Extension	5 × 30
Calf Raise	5 × 25
Front Calf Raise	5 × 25
Lunge	4 × 25
Leg Stretching	2 × 20
Calf Stretching	2 × 20
Triceps Pushdown	2 × 15
Lateral Raise	2 × 15
Bent-Over Lateral Raise	2 × 15
Side Bend	4 × 25
Sit-Up	4 × 25
Hyperextension	4 × 25
Jumping Rope—Up to 10 minutes	

Surfing

Surfing, which once was exclusively the sport of Hawaiian kings, has now attracted more than 2 million enthusiasts around the world. Learning the art of balance and relaxation needed to control the slippery board depends a great deal on the strength of your leg muscles. If they are not strong enough, you will be forced to pivot your hips and upper body, causing delayed turns. Delays in reaction time will limit your feeling of confidence in controlling the board. You also must have strong arm muscles to match the speed of the waves as you paddle just ahead of the onrushing water toward shore.

Building endurance and stamina is particularly important in a big surf when the interval between waves is between 13 and 19 seconds. If you should fall off the board, this gives you only 20 seconds to surface before the next wave breaks over you. The following routine will strengthen your legs and shoulders and increase the vital capacity of your lungs.

Squat	3 × 20
Leg Extension	3 × 20
Pulldown	3 × 15
Bench Press	3 × 15
Triceps Pushdown	3 × 15
Calf Raise	5 × 15

Tennis

A good weight training program builds a reserve of strength that can be as important as good strokes for developing your match-winning skills to the maximum. The staying power needed to keep the ball in play without getting tired will give you that extra edge to defeat those who are equal to you in ability but lack your fitness.

For the most part tennis players have been introduced to bodybuilding after an injury, such as having the anterior cruciate ligament, which keeps the knee from slipping, give way. By training the quadriceps and hamstring muscles, athletes have often built more strength on the injured side than on the uninjured one.

Leg Extensions are the best exercises to help prevent knee injuries. In addition, they equalize imbalances so your weight is planted solidly prior to your stroke, giving you the advantage of having a strong hitting foundation. Wrist Curls will strengthen your grip, add power to your stroke (off either side), and help prevent tennis elbow.

Lunge	2 × 20
Leg Extension	4 × 25
Calf Raise	2 × 20
Front Calf Raise	2 × 20
Barbell Rowing	2 × 10
One-Arm Rowing	2 × 10
Bent-Over Lateral Raise	2 × 10
Lateral Raise	2 × 10
Triceps Pushdown	2 × 10
Wrist Curl	2 × 10
Abdominal Training—the next 2 exercises are done in rotation.	
Sit-Up	4 × 25
Leg Raise	4 × 25
Hamstring Stretch	1 × 5
Calf Stretching	1 × 5
Side Bend	1 × 5

Volleyball

Like basketball, this sport calls for endurance and explosive movements when you spike the ball over the net. Unless players are in top physical shape, their muscles will tire and fail to respond properly during prolonged competition. For example, a good jumper with poor endurance will contact the ball 30 inches above the net during warm-ups, but only 20 inches during the fifth game of a match.

These exercises will increase the height of vertical jumps and build the ability to sustain maximum efforts throughout long matches and tournaments. Also emphasized are exercises for backcourt players whose low squatting position tends to sap vital leg strength unless their muscles are thoroughly conditioned. Do not neglect exercises for the abdominal muscles and to a lesser degree the back muscles because they play a large part in a player's spiking action.

Bear in mind that nothing hinders endurance for any sport as much as being overweight. When a volleyball player is 10 pounds overweight he must jump and lift those 10 extra pounds hundreds of times during a match.

Lunge	3 × 20
Squat	2 × 20
Leg Extension	3 × 25
Pulldown	3 × 15
Lateral Raise	3 × 10
Side Bend	2 × 10
Sit-Up	3 × 25
Leg Raise	3 × 25
Running	2–3 miles

Wrestling

Although wrestling is an instinctive sport that seems to come naturally, it is necessary to train for all the bulk and power you can effectively use. Bruno San Martino trained with weights from the beginning of his wrestling career. In all probability he could have become a champion performer in powerlifting. One of his most sensational feats performed in the wrestling ring was lifting "Haystacks" Calhoun—who stood 6'4" and weighed 641 pounds—off his feet and hurling him to the mat! Certainly weight training has been a definite asset to San Martino and added to the public's enjoyment of wrestling matches. This program includes all three powerlifting exercises, and I suggest that you perform each one with maximum weight.

Squat	4 × 10
Leg Press	4 × 10
Deadlift	4 × 5
Bench Press	4 × 10
Barbell Rowing	4 × 10
Triceps Pushdown	5 × 10
Barbell Curl	4 × 8
Standing Press	3 × 10
Presses behind Neck	3 × 10
Lateral Raise	4 × 10
Wrist Curl	4 × 10

Seven

How to Handle Exercise Injuries

Many men plan their lives, business activities, and family finances with great care, yet when it comes to exercising, a great number give little thought to preparing the body for additional exertion to which they are unaccustomed. Remember, bodybuilding is a mental as well as physical achievement. Knowing which factors are likely to cause injury is the best way to prevent them.

Prevention

Poor concentration is one of the most common causes of injury. When your mind wanders you are liable to pick up a heavier weight and begin training without full concentration, leaving yourself prone to injury. It is impossible to focus on good form when talking to others. This lack of concentration causes movements to become jerky, and if the body is thrown awkwardly in completing a movement, there's a good chance of sustaining a painful injury. By keeping a steadfast focus on your equipment and body, each repetition can be done in strict form, smoothly and rhythmically. Having this control, you are less likely to pull muscles or otherwise injure yourself.

Muscles become more contracted with weight training; therefore, they need to be stretched before and after training. A hard workout engenders microscopic muscle damage. If not allowed time to heal, the muscles shorten and become liable to tearing, unless flexibility is restored by stretching. Tight hamstring muscles will contribute to lower back pain, so they should be stretched daily.

Warming up, like stretching, is one of the best ways to prevent injury. Since the synovial fluid around the joints acts as a lubricant, it must be circulating before heavy training is begun. In cooler weather it is important to warm up for a longer period of time. Do some light exercise before doing anything heavy, and if you must include weights as part of the warm-up, make them dumbbell weights.

As mentioned above, muscle fibers are broken down or torn slightly during heavy training. Healing takes place during the day of rest between workouts, provided enough protein is in the body to repair the tissues. Lack of sufficient protein in the diet will cause a slow rate of repair that will keep you from progressing on the training program. A further elaboration on the importance of protein is given in the section on nutrition.

A mineral deficiency can cause a separation of muscles and ligaments that attach to the bones. Calcium and magnesium are needed for muscle movement. If calcium is lacking, muscles will begin to contract and spasm. Magnesium regulates the conversion of carbohydrates to energy. A shortage of potassium in your system may cause weakness and a tired feeling for an extended period of time. During heavy training, potassium is released into the bloodstream by the muscles to keep them from overheating. As blood vessels widen, the flow of blood is increased and heat is drawn away from the muscles. The potassium is then excreted from the body by sweat and urine. Heavy training and a high-protein diet will increase the body's requirements for calcium, magnesium, and potassium.

Overtraining generates a tendency to ignore warning signals sent out by the body, such as persistent pain in bones, muscles, and joints. This can lead to serious injuries. Those who are highly competitive tend to ignore pain since they are driven by a need to reach goals that are sometimes unrealistic. Common signs of overtraining are a limited span of concentration, fatigue, lack of a pump, lowered resistance to infection or colds, lowered desire to train, and more than the usual aches and pains during a workout.

Throughout the training programs I have recommended that the exercises be followed in the sequence given. Incorrect training causes an imbalance in the body. Every muscle that moves a limb in one direction has an opposing muscle to move it another direction. So some muscle groups need to be trained more and others less, or the entire structure is thrown out of balance. If one muscle is far stronger than the other, it can overpower and damage the weaker one.

In conclusion, never force yourself to do an exercise because everyone in the gym does it as a matter of course. Remember, each body is different. If something works for 10 or 20 other guys, it may not work for you. It may, in fact, actually cause harm. When a piece of equipment feels uncomfortable, don't use it. Always tune in to your own body and learn to distinguish what makes you feel better.

Causes of Injuries

I find it important to preface this section by recommending that you consult a doctor of chiropractic for sports injuries. While your family doctor is usually excellent for diagnosing and treating illness, his knowledge of sports injuries may be limited. His prescription for a painkiller, and his advice to take it easy for a while, may be the worst treatment for your particular problem. Doctors of chiropractic, however, center the majority of their studies around body mechanics (kinesiology) and nutrition, the two areas of medicine that most often play major roles in sports injuries.

About the most common injuries are muscle strains and sprained ligaments, which cause the spinal vertebrae to move out of position and slightly displace the bones. Commonly called a *pinched nerve*, this means the nerve supply from the brain and spinal cord to an organ or extremity has been diminished by existing pressure on a particular nerve or group of them. At our Chiropractic Center we have found pinched nerves especially common among powerlifters and bodybuilders. At times certain exercises such as Squats need to be eliminated. When the normal nerve function is restored, however, the symptoms are usually reversible and the body returns to normal.

Types of Injury

The following discussion of injuries by body part will give you an insight into their usual causes and means of prevention.

Knee

One of the most complicated articulations of the body is the knee. Because this joint is held together by ligaments, it is not particularly stable. It can be injured in at least four places: the kneecap tendons, the cartilages, the ligaments, and the muscles around the knee. Its only natural movement is bending forward, so squatting with your feet too far apart or with your toes pointed too far in or out can easily

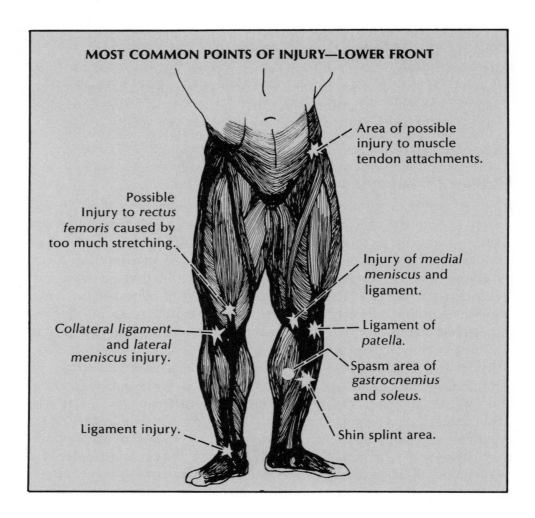

MOST COMMON POINTS OF INJURY—LOWER FRONT

Area of possible injury to muscle tendon attachments.

Possible Injury to *rectus femoris* caused by too much stretching.

Injury of *medial meniscus* and ligament.

Collateral ligament and *lateral meniscus* injury.

Ligament of *patella.*

Spasm area of *gastrocnemius* and *soleus.*

Ligament injury.

Shin splint area.

cause knee problems. Tight hamstring muscles also will contribute to knee problems; therefore, the importance of stretching the hamstring muscles daily cannot be overemphasized. If you have a knee injury, immediately have it checked by a physician since these injuries can develop into more serious problems.

Ankle

Injuries to the ankle are usually caused by keeping the ankle stiff and the calf muscles too tight during strenuous activity. The most effective exercise for preventing ankle injuries is to stand with the ball of your foot on a block of wood or on the lowest step of a staircase and let your heels drop down off the block of wood or stair step to stretch for one minute.

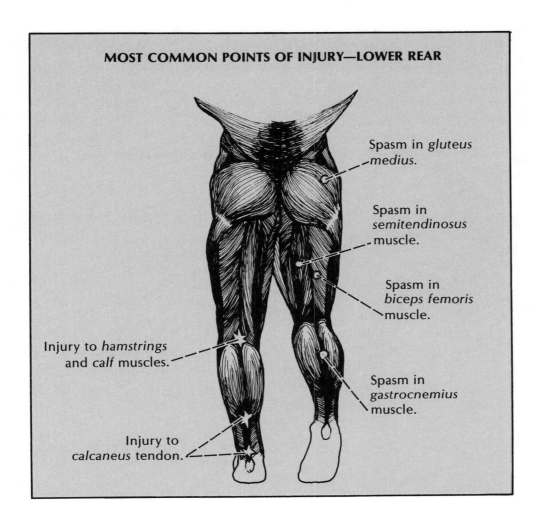

MOST COMMON POINTS OF INJURY—LOWER REAR

Spasm in *gluteus medius.*

Spasm in *semitendinosus* muscle.

Spasm in *biceps femoris* muscle.

Spasm in *gastrocnemius* muscle.

Injury to *hamstrings* and *calf* muscles.

Injury to *calcaneus* tendon.

Femur

The head of the femur forms a deep ball-and-socket joint with the pelvis, making it a stable joint. Problems will develop if you squat with the toes pointed too far in or out or if you do split-type exercises for stretching inner thigh muscles. Injuries to the femur joints should be treated by a doctor of chiropractic. There are no effective treatments for slight displacements other than adjustments with kinesiology to strengthen muscles around the femur.

Middle Back

This area is easily affected by Presses and T-Bar Rowing because such exercises stress the ribs attached to the vertebral bodies. When the ribs are moved slightly out of position a stabbing pain can ensue,

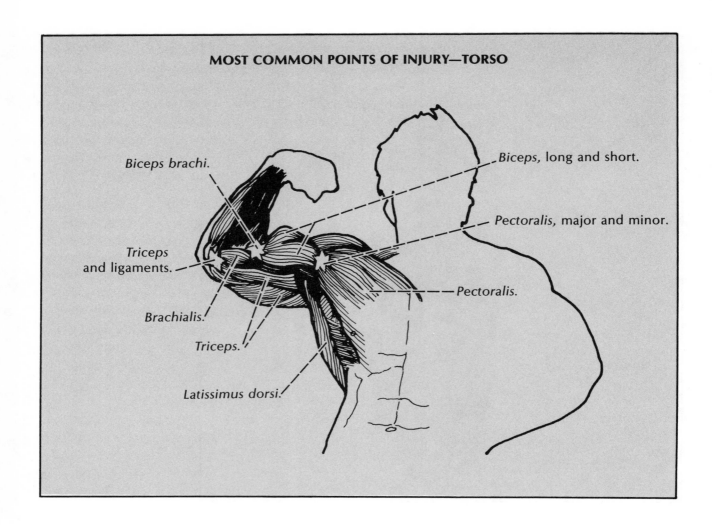

MOST COMMON POINTS OF INJURY—TORSO

Biceps brachi.

Biceps, long and short.

Triceps and ligaments.

Pectoralis, major and minor.

Brachialis.

Pectoralis.

Triceps.

Latissimus dorsi.

especially when moving in a certain direction, coughing, or sneezing. Sometimes One-Arm Rowing is helpful with this problem, but most often chiropractic care is needed for effective treatment.

Lower Back

Many bodybuilders' problems with the lower back are caused by Straight-Leg Sit-Ups, Roman Chair Sit-Ups, Squats, Deadlifts, Presses, and sleeping on your stomach. All the training programs in this book were designed to prevent these problems. Here again I call your attention to the importance of using correct form when training and avoiding any jerking movements.

Stretching the hamstring muscles is essential for individuals who have sustained lower back injuries. Other corrective exercises are Standing Side Bends; lying on your back and pulling one knee to the chest; or lying on the floor with bent knees and holding your arms around the knees while rocking back and forth.

If you have injured the lower back, avoid all Sit-Ups, Press exercises, and Deadlifts until completely recovered. A doctor who is familiar with sports should be consulted before continuing these exercises.

Shoulder

Most injuries to the shoulders are caused by Reverse Curls, which, along with Presses, should be eliminated from your program until the shoulder injury heals. Since the shoulder joint is supported by muscles, I have emphasized Bent-Over Lateral Raises, which are the best exercise for preventing shoulder injuries.

Neck

Bodybuilders may have problems in this area due to some form of muscular imbalance. Usually the trapezius muscle is strong while the anterior neck muscles are weak. Minor problems can be aggravated by doing presses or holding your hands behind the neck for Sit-Ups. Instead, place your hands on your chest for the Sit-Ups, and the neck flexors will be exercised during the process of moving your head up and down.

Elbows

Due to an imbalance between the biceps and triceps muscles in the upper arm, problems with the elbows sometimes occur. The triceps are long muscles that usually are weaker than the biceps; therefore, they must be worked harder to keep them in balance with the biceps. Because most men tend to underwork the triceps, I have recommended more sets for them than for the biceps. Those who decide to intensify their training for the biceps should also increase work on the triceps to keep both sets balanced.

Wrist

Most wrist problems are caused by an imbalance of the forearm muscles or by flexing the hand too far back toward the elbow. These injuries can usually be corrected by doing Hanging Wrist Curls, which help balance the forearm muscles.

Muscle Soreness

Even those in top physical shape can develop soreness in muscles not often used. It usually sets in 8–24 hours after a workout and lasts about three to five hours. If it persists, however, this may indicate a deficiency of vitamin C.

Muscle Spasm

A spasm, which can last for several days, is caused by involuntary contractions of muscles. At times nerve pressure and lack of circulation compound the problem. Common remedies include applications of ice or moist heat on the area; increasing intake of minerals, particularly calcium; and stretching the muscles around the affected area.

Muscle Cramps

A muscle cramp is a painful and sustained contraction of all the fibers in a muscle, lasting for a few seconds or several hours. It is usually caused by nerve pressure and/or deficiencies in calcium, magnesium, and potassium.

Sprain

When some of the fibers of a ligament are torn it is referred to as a *sprain*. Sprains can be caused by overstretching ligaments while under stress or by twisting too far in areas around the joints and causing a partial tearing of the fibers. If you incur a sprain, immediately stop exercising the area or you will aggravate the injury and cause complications. You must see a physician and rest the injured area. In the majority of cases the ligament reattaches itself by laying down new cells.

Strain

These injuries usually occur where the tendon attaches to the bone. Although muscles and tendons are integral units, tendons are more susceptible to injury since they have a smaller cross section than muscles. Because the area over which force is distributed in tendons is limited, they are more liable to strain than muscles. Athletes taking steroid drugs and thyroid medications are more prone to muscle tendon injuries because drugs create mineral imbalances.

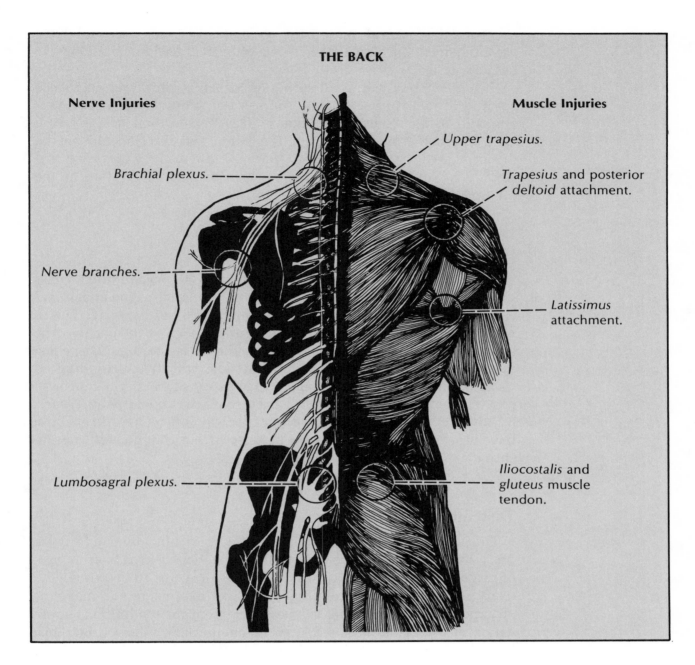

THE BACK

Nerve Injuries

Muscle Injuries

Upper trapesius.

Brachial plexus.

Trapesius and posterior *deltoid* attachment.

Nerve branches.

Latissimus attachment.

Lumbosagral plexus.

Iliocostalis and *gluteus* muscle tendon.

Bursitis

This condition gets its name from the bursas, saclike cavities containing synovial fluids to protect the joints from rubbing together. When this tissue becomes inflamed or calcium deposits form, bursitis results. The most commonly inflamed areas are the knee, elbow, and shoulder joints. Habitually using one arm more than another as required by baseball, golf, and tennis can lead to bursitis. The problem can be greatly compounded by training on machines, restricting the natural movement of joints. For this reason I have recommended working with free weights that accommodate to your body structure.

If you have bursitis, avoid eating citrus fruits while training, since citric acid neutralizes synovial fluid in the joints. Most experts recommend using ice on the inflamed area rather than heat because heat increases inflammation of the joint. The fluid should not be drained except in severe cases because the body will produce a similar quantity to replace the amount drained. Elevation of the inflamed area is also helpful.

Hernia

A hernia is an abnormal protrusion of a bodily organ into a canal or opening. Commonly, hernias are closely related to the abdominal cavity and frequently contain a portion of the digestive tract. This is caused by a weakening of the structures supporting the organs. The most common type among male bodybuilders is the inguinal hernia in the groin, occurring when intraabdominal structures descend through the canal. Occasionally, perhaps due to a slight defect in construction of the canal or from excessive intraabdominal pressure, a "knuckle" of the intestine may work its way into an aperture. If you have a hernia, get medical care because lifting weights will complicate it.

Tendinitis

This is an inflammation causing the fibers within a tendon to swell. Most often this results from overusing a particular area or from lack of circulation in the area. Because the pain seems to decrease with exercise, many athletes continue playing or exercising and make the situation worse. I find that the best treatment for tendinitis is application of ice to the inflamed area for one minute, followed by moist heat for 5 minutes. This treatment should be followed twice daily, and training should be avoided until the injury is fully healed.

Fractures

A fracture is a break, rupture, or crack in a bone. If the continuity of the bone is broken or severed, it is a complete fracture. When the bone is cracked but not separated, it is a stress fracture. Usually, complete fractures are the most painful because the jagged edges of the separated bones have a supply of nerves that rub against each other and the surrounding tissue, causing extreme pain. If you suspect that you have fractured a bone, see your physician immediately for an examination of the injured area and x-rays to determine the extent of damage. Never attempt to treat fractures yourself. I have found minerals valuable in reducing the healing time of fractures.

Treating Injuries

The most common injuries to bodybuilders are strains, sprains, tendon tears, cramps, and hernias. Placing an ice pack or ice cube directly over the area of pain will help reduce any swelling and inflammation. Ice decreases bleeding from injured blood vessels by causing them to contract. When a quantity of blood collects in a wound it takes longer to heal. In addition, you can elevate the injured area so the force of gravity will help drain excess fluid.

Don't attempt to diagnose yourself and don't follow the advice of anyone in a gym. Most injuries require professional care. You should seek the advice of a doctor who specializes in sports injuries and understands the mechanism of different exercises. Although a good number of injuries heal by themselves, if some are left untreated, they could develop into serious problems.

As previously mentioned, doctors of chiropractic are excellent for sports injuries not requiring surgery, since they are expert in structural alignment, body mechanics, and corrective exercises. If the injury seems like a muscle, tendon, or ligamental tear or a bone fracture, however, see a medical doctor or orthopedic surgeon immediately. In many cases you will be able to continue training, but your program will need some revision.

Additional guidelines for home treatment of sports injuries follow.

1. Use moist heat on chronic muscle spasms.
2. Do stretching exercises for tight muscles.
3. Apply pressure at the center of a spasm to relax the muscles.
4. Whenever the pain is severe, stop training immediately and send for medical help.

Exercises that Cause Injury

Many exercises commonly done in gyms and health spas are a total waste of time, but even worse, some can cause permanent damage. For example, one of the most common is a waist-twisting exercise done by holding a pole across the shoulders and twisting the upper body from right to left. Even without the pole, this exercise can cause lower back strains. Yet, it would be a rare occasion to enter a gym or health club without seeing a number of people doing this exercise in the mistaken belief that they are reducing fat deposits around the waist.

I do not know who invented this exercise or the reason millions sincerely believe in its effectiveness. However, with my vast experience as a doctor and professional athlete, I know that this exercise can cause permanent damage to the lower back lumbar area when done repeatedly. To be specific, it can damage the sagittal facets, vertical segments located in the lumbar area of the spine. These segments are made to bend forward. When the waist-twisting exercise is done with a pole lodged across the shoulders, the body is forced to twist up to 50 degrees, as opposed to its normal flexion of 30 degrees. Forcing the body to twist beyond its normal capacity can cause degeneration of a thin pad located between the sagittal facets and may also result in early arthritis problems of the lower back.

Spinal problems can also be caused by a twister apparatus mounted on casters. You will always find several people using these devices, energetically swiveling the lower part of the body from right to left. This exercise may seem impressive, and the people may seem to know exactly what they are doing, however, swiveling on this apparatus does not reduce fat around the waist or tone the hips and thighs. On the contrary, it produces no positive results but can be highly effective in causing back muscles to contract and spasm.

Another piece of equipment that should never be used is the Roman chair. This also strains the lower spinal region, lumbar area, and the pelvis rather than works the stomach muscles.

Many traditional stomach exercises you are accustomed to doing may not be found in this book since they cause problems in the hip and lower portion of the spine. When done incorrectly, Sit-Ups cause the iliopsoas muscles, attached to the lumbar vertebrae and disks, to spasm. When this occurs the vertebrae are moved out of alignment and the bone presses on the nerve root, causing a pinched nerve. The Sit-Ups I developed for every program in this book are founded on my bodybuilding knowledge and research in body mechanics. Each exercise for the stomach area will protect the spine while strengthening and toning the stomach muscles.

Keep in mind that the body tries to maintain balance and equilibrium no matter what happens. This tendency applies to the body's structure as well as its organs. An imbalance in one area will immediately cause stress in another that is trying to carry a heavier load, resulting in your having two problems where previously you had only one. Therefore, be aware of certain exercises routinely given to every newcomer, particularly in health spas. Do not assume that 20 people leaping up and down doing an exercise such as Jumping Jacks is proof positive that it is beneficial to your well-being. Jumping Jacks, Bench Squats, Headstands, and Side Bends with weights can cause body imbalances. All are of highly questionable benefit and, if done repeatedly, can make you susceptible to other injuries.

Eight

Shaping Up Your Lifestyle

As important as the physical components of your lifestyle—nutrition, exercise, etc.—are the mental, emotional, and environmental aspects, as well as the patterns and habits you exhibit in your daily life. To shape up in the fullest sense you must manage your entire life well. In this chapter I will identify and discuss some of the ways you can round out your fitness program: reducing stress, avoiding drugs, controlling your environment, and taking care of yourself by anticipating health hazards.

Stress Reduction

The only people I know who are free of stress live in Sardinia, an island off the coast of Italy where I was born. Here the people live simply and are closely rooted to the earth, so they have less to worry about. In contrast, Americans tend to concern themselves with 50 different problems, which they try to solve successfully in the course of one day.

In Sardinia the prime concern is making a living to provide food for the family. Sardinians rarely worry about anything else or suffer from tension because there is no crime and family problems are rare. Usually they live in their own homes, happily tending their own gardens and growing their own food. If there is illness in the family or some other worry, the people in Sardinia—and this includes me— lose their appetite and stop eating.

The contrary situation exists in the United States, where stress triggers an eating binge for most people. "I'm having an anxiety attack" is the explanation often given when someone gobbles up a candy bar or polishes off a slice of chocolate cake topped with ice cream. As I see it, these people are using stress, anxiety, or worry as an excuse to eat. I find this difficult to understand because stress causes my digestive juices to stop secreting and cuts down my appetite. Therefore, I've been led to conclude that many people either formed a habit of equating stress with eating or were trained to eat when under stress. The problem seems to stem from environmental factors rather than being inherent.

Many times stress is caused by problems that seem to have no immediate solution. One way to relieve the resultant anxiety is to learn to think through your problems logically, evaluate possible solutions, and then set the problems aside. For instance, your car could break down one evening when all the repair shops are closed. You could bring on a good case of frazzled nerves by running the problem around and around in your head instead of telling yourself that you can do nothing until the following morning. Simply put the problem aside and pick it up again the next day by getting a mechanic who can fix the car and get you on the road again.

If this kind of talking to yourself does not relieve the stress, then go to the gym and have a good workout. Research has proven that vigorous exercise is the best antidote for nervous and emotional stress, working far better than tranquilizers or sedatives. A test conducted with men 50 years old and older proved that a 15-minute walk reduced neuromuscular tension more effectively than any tranquilizer. If repeated and regular, exercise will also condition the stress adaption mechanisms of the body, which provide a degree of protection against emotional stress. The physically fit individual has the advantage of a greater adrenal reserve with larger amounts of steroids available to counter prolonged tension.

Foods that Cause Stress

Certain types of food will also cause stress. One of the most common is refined sugar, which causes a vitamin B_{12} deficiency and lowers the mineral content in the body. This makes people hyperactive, with the end result being a high degree of nervousness, which places stress on the entire body. A similar problem is encountered by drinking large amounts of coffee because it acts on the brain and central nervous system. If taken in excess, caffeine can induce a certain degree of disorientation and suppress the natural warning signals induced by fatigue, especially if the individual is physically under par. In addition, the chemicals used in processing coffee and decaffeinated coffee can be toxic when consumed in large amounts.

Smoking

Another common stress-causing agent is cigarette smoking because physiologically nicotine stimulates the sympathetic nervous system. Many people smoke for the purpose of relaxation that may last 5–10 minutes, but directly afterward they get nervous again and light up another cigarette. This causes a jagged up-and-down pattern of relaxing and getting hyperactive, which is detrimental to the normal functioning of the body and places it under constant stress.

Sleeping

In some instances an individual's sleeping habits can cause stress. Many people have insomnia because they disrupt their sleep cycle by taking naps when watching television and then have difficulty falling asleep at bedtime. They lie in bed worrying about their inability to sleep, which in turn triggers other worries concerning business, family, or personal behavior. In time they form a habit of worrying instead of sleeping every time their head touches the pillow at night. Ideally, one should sleep a minimum of seven hours and a maximum of eight, depending on the individual. Excessive sleep, on the other hand, may indicate a desire to escape from situations or problems that should be corrected.

Blood Pressure

If you feel you are under constant stress, consider having tests taken to determine food allergies and others to check levels of fatty substances in the blood. A stressful situation puts the nervous system on alert and sends messages to the brain, which in turn initiates an increase in the level of triglycerides and cholesterol in the bloodstream. This causes a tensing of muscles, rapid pulse, fast breathing, and an increase in blood pressure. If you suffer chronic stress, you should also have a physical examination to check your blood pressure and pulse rate according to how you exercise. If your normal level is 120 over 80, it should drop about 10 points after a few minutes of working out. Those exercising regularly usually have a blood pressure level 10 percent lower than that of individuals who are sedentary.

Because your blood pressure is an important guide in determining the existence of certain physical problems, I will briefly explain the dynamics of its highs and lows. Your blood pressure is taken to establish the existing pressure in the large arteries at the height of the pulse rate. The highest point is the *systolic* pressure, the force of the blood being pumped when the heart is contracted. The *diastolic*, or lower, reading is reached when the heart is relaxed. Moderate exercise may not influence the systolic pressure; however, it will rise when exercise becomes strenuous, such as in going upstairs, running, or training with little rest between sets. At night, when asleep, the lowest point of pressure is reached.

Many people worry when their systolic blood pressure is above 120, believing themselves in precarious physical condition because a normal reading is 120 over 80. They should realize that a reading of 130 over 90 is also normal. However, 130 over 80 would signal a problem because of the 50-point difference between the systolic and diastolic pressures. This is the difference that would concern your doctor.

Of course, blood pressure levels will vary during the day and from day to day. There are slight changes according to age, sex, altitude (mountains or sea level), and muscular development. In general, the reading is 5–10 points lower in women than in men. Fatigue, business pressures, and other emotional stimuli can cause the arterioles to constrict by way of the nervous system. Another fact to consider is body weight: with every 10 extra pounds the blood pressure level can increase five points. Also, the level will increase as you become older. Until 25 or 30 the normal level may be 120 over 80; then it increases one point every two years without being a cause for alarm.

Research has proven exercise one of the most effective ways to control high blood pressure. After a training program the diastolic pressure is lower, the systolic pressure increases less during exercise, and elasticity of the small arteries is increased. When exercising, veins in the mass of body muscles are affected by contraction and relaxation. For example, veins in the legs are squeezed or "milked" each time the leg muscles contract, so the blood in them is forced in the direction of the heart. After exercise there is also an increase in the number of red blood cells in the circulatory system due to the development of red marrow in the bones.

Heart Rate

Research has shown that running and weightlifting both increase the size of the heart, causing it to become stronger, just like any muscle that is used often. However, only weightlifters develop hearts with thicker and stronger walls, which lowers the resting heart rate

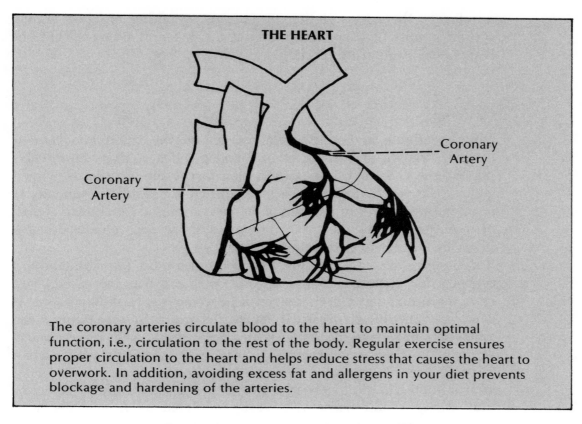

THE HEART

Coronary Artery

Coronary Artery

The coronary arteries circulate blood to the heart to maintain optimal function, i.e., circulation to the rest of the body. Regular exercise ensures proper circulation to the heart and helps reduce stress that causes the heart to overwork. In addition, avoiding excess fat and allergens in your diet prevents blockage and hardening of the arteries.

an'd makes it more efficient. The stroke volume is increased so that fewer heartbeats are required for a given cardiac output, making the heart rate and blood pressure return more rapidly to normal after activity. For instance, the average heart rate of individuals is 72 beats per minute, but for those lifting weights it drops to 60 beats. Many weightlifters who are not overweight have heart rates of 55–65 beats per minute.

Keep in mind that every 10 pounds of fat causes the heart rate to increase by about 5 beats. On the other hand, if the weight gain is purely muscular, your heart rate most likely will remain the same or even decrease. The key to gaining maximum heart improvement with weight training is to rest as little as possible between sets and to go from one exercise to another without stopping.

Drugs and Other Harmful Substances

Our fast-paced society has become dependent on the instant gratification of drugs to promote better performance, depress anxiety, and make relaxation come easily. Ignored is the fact that drugs have detrimental effects on physiological functioning and are toxic to the body. Most of them have a direct effect on muscle fibers. They counteract the accumulation of fatigue by acting on the nervous system, supply fuel for muscular contractions, and act on the cardio-respiratory regulating mechanism.

Caffeine

Both caffeine and amphetamines act on the brain and central nervous system, increasing mental and physical activity and delaying fatigue. This artificial stimulation forces the body to use emergency reserves that should be replenished by rest. The amount of pure caffeine found in one cup of coffee is minimal (about one-eighth of a teaspoon), yet the total amount in three cups equals dosages given by doctors to stimulate the heart.

The effects of drinking coffee can be felt almost immediately and continue for a number of hours. Coffee may cause an increased heart rate, insomnia, and a high degree of nervousness. In the long term it can raise the blood pressure, cause the heart to race, injure the pancreas, and make diabetes and hypoglycemia worse. Since it also retards the digestive process by inhibiting secretion of digestive juices, it can cause peptic ulcers. Yet here in America we drink approximately half of the coffee grown in the world. I have no doubt that others would become as easily addicted as Americans, who drink an average of three cups daily, except coffee is very expensive and the majority of people worldwide cannot afford to indulge themselves.

Those hoping to circumvent the problem by drinking decaffeinated coffee should be aware that the caffeine is removed by using methylene chloride, a solvent that can cause cancer when taken extensively. Recently a process using steam to remove caffeine from coffee without leaving a dangerous residue like methylene chloride was developed in Switzerland. However, this product is high-priced and not normally stocked in most markets. Since espresso is also produced by steaming, a great deal of the caffeine is dissipated along with the steam, making it safer to drink than regular coffee, which is perked or kept hot for long hours in coffee shops and restaurants. Because espresso is steamed quickly under pressure, it is low in acid as well as caffeine.

Remember that caffeine travels very quickly to the bloodstream and causes very fast changes in the body, including dilating the blood vessels and causing a 10 percent increase in the metabolic rate. It also increases the output of stomach acid in the urine, and the excretion of magnesium is more than quadrupled. A magnesium deficiency causes nervousness, tension, and hangover jitters similar to those brought on after a night of drinking heavily. The lethal dose of caffeine is about 10 thousand milligrams, or about 100 cups of coffee.

Many individuals do not realize caffeine is also found in tea, soft drinks, chocolate, and a number of prescription drugs taken for headaches. Tea, with the exception of herb teas labeled "no caffeine," contains almost as much caffeine as coffee. A great deal of caffeine is found in prescription drugs such as Anacin, Excedrin, Midol, and aspirin. And, of course, the stay-alert tablets such as No-Doz that are available in drugstores are almost all caffeine. There are significant amounts in chocolate beverages, milk chocolate, and baking chocolate. Caffeine is contained in more than half of the soft drinks available. However, the following are caffeine-free: 7-Up, Pepsi-Free, Diet Sunkist, Canada Dry Ginger Ale, RC 100, Sunkist, Fresca, and Sprite.

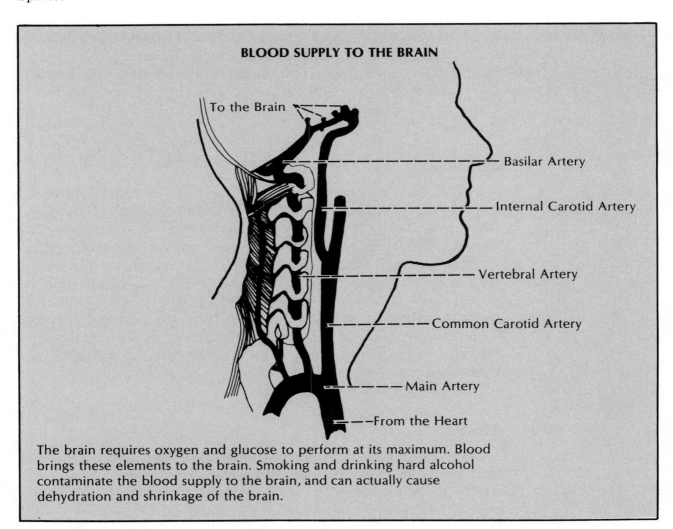

BLOOD SUPPLY TO THE BRAIN

To the Brain

Basilar Artery

Internal Carotid Artery

Vertebral Artery

Common Carotid Artery

Main Artery

From the Heart

The brain requires oxygen and glucose to perform at its maximum. Blood brings these elements to the brain. Smoking and drinking hard alcohol contaminate the blood supply to the brain, and can actually cause dehydration and shrinkage of the brain.

Cigarettes

On-every pack of cigarettes is found the warning, "The Surgeon General has determined that cigarette smoking is dangerous to your health." Unfortunately, smokers have a tendency to blot this warning from their consciousness. I find it difficult to understand why they ignore the well-publicized connection between smoking and lung and bladder cancer, chronic bronchitis, and emphysema. Physiologically, nicotine stimulates the sympathetic nervous system and triggers overconsumption of oxygen by the heart, making it a related cause of heart disease. Researchers at the University of Massachusetts have recently estimated that smoking a pack and a half a day is the yearly equivalent of radiation doses from 300 x-rays. It will also increase the level of certain triglycerides and cholesterol, and every cigarette destroys 15–25 milligrams of vitamin C, making the smoker more susceptible to bacterial infections and colds.

There is evidence to suggest that inactive smokers are three times more likely to suffer a heart attack than smokers who are moderately active. And the active smoker has a better chance of surviving a heart attack than the nonactive smoker. Many adults who participate in regular exercise programs have drastically reduced smoking or eliminated it altogether.

Marijuana

If you plan on switching to marijuana in an effort to give up cigarettes, you will be worse off. For example, one joint of marijuana contains as much tar as 100 regular cigarettes, and the body retains 30 percent of its active agents for a week. No other drugs or medication are known to linger in the body for this length of time. Of the portion remaining, 70 percent is retained in the body longer than the second week. The main damage occurs to the brain and autonomic nervous system, which alters all the body controls and thinking centers, causing atrophy of the brain and muscles if individuals are heavy users. In addition, it is known to cause greater damage to the lungs than cigarettes.

Alcohol

In my experience most native Italians do not drink wine, beer, or cordials because of psychological problems, boredom, or unsociability. To them, a glass of wine with a meal is as natural as having a slice of bread, a piece of fruit, or a green salad. Wine is not singled out to provide relief from stress but to accompany a good meal and add a touch of elegance to hospitality, such as the small thimbleful of anisette ordinarily served to guests.

When hard alcohol is used in an effort to cope with problems, mask conflicts, or escape reality, it becomes a problem. Degenerative diseases of the liver, heart, and blood vessels are likely to occur in heavy drinkers. Excessive intake of alcohol hastens damage to the brain because it cuts off the supply of oxygen, killing a large number of brain cells. Since brain cells do not multiply, they are irreplaceable. Research has shown that people who drank excessively for 25 or more years had brains that were four pounds smaller than normal size. Also, in blocking out certain thought processes over a period of time, alcohol produces varying degrees of disintegration of the nervous system.

If possible, it is important to avoid hard alcohol. However, I recommend having a glass of wine or beer during lunch or dinner since they are both low in alcohol. It has been reported that beer is extremely beneficial for lactating mothers, and wine contains more than 300 enzymes that help to digest food.

Salt Pills and Diuretics

The fluid in and around the body cells has a delicate sodium/potassium balance that is upset by diuretics and salt pills. Sweating causes you to lose proportionately more water than salt, leaving a higher level of sodium in the bloodstream. By taking salt tablets you elevate that level even more. Your blood thickens and is more likely to clot with a heavy concentration of salt in the bloodstream. Clots may cause strokes, heart attacks, and kidney failure. When your body needs extra salt, you will begin craving food containing it. Even for a healthy person, having excess salt is more dangerous than not having enough.

Diuretics also cause potassium to be excreted, resulting in a mineral imbalance with deficiencies of magnesium, B vitamins, and many other nutrients. Potassium and magnesium are vital in helping prevent heart attacks, and a lack of these minerals allows clots to form in the heart and brain. Loss of vitamin B and pantothenic acid can cause decreased circulation, degeneration of the heart muscles, and excessive excretion of iodine.

Starch Blockers

The latest "miracle" for dieters is the antistarch pills. Sold under a variety of names, these starch stoppers are advertised as a way to eat bread, pasta, and other starches without concern for their caloric content. The active ingredient in these pills is a kidney bean extract formulated to block the enzyme action that processes starch in the digestive process.

Research done on animals has shown that these antistarch pills could permanently damage the pancreas. When enzyme production is inhibited the pancreas tries to overcompensate by producing more of the enzymes and ends up working itself to death.

Controlling Your Environment

Today's environment can be a hostile one to the human body. And while you can never control your surroundings completely, you can make certain efforts to minimize hazards to your health.

Air Purity

Nothing is more vitalizing than pure, fresh air. Yet most of the time we breathe air that is either warmed or cooled by machines in the office, at home, in planes, restaurants, and our cars. Air conditioning seems to cause the most damage because it not only alters the temperature but also changes the amount of oxygen in the atmosphere.

By drawing moisture from the environment, air conditioning contributes to the cause of many viral infections that are anaerobic, infecting the body when it receives the least amount of oxygen. For example, when you have a cold, viruses become lodged in the sinus areas, trachea, and esophagus. One of the best-known remedies for a virus cold is inhalation of hot steam. Being rich in oxygen, it penetrates the pockets of the mouth, sinuses, and nose.

Air conditioning has the opposite effect, decreasing the flow of oxygen to these areas, where the resultant dryness causes the virus to increase and multiply. For these reasons air conditioning should be used only when absolutely necessary, especially in your car.

Those who work in centrally air-conditioned offices can help their bodies retain a natural level of moisture by placing a large container of water close to the air flow vent and drinking one glass of water every hour.

Running and Exercising Environment

Whenever possible, try to exercise in the sunlight where the air is clean. It has been found that the ultraviolet rays of the sun, when combined with increased body temperature, reduce blood pressure as well as cholesterol and triglyceride levels that are above normal. When it is necessary to work out at the gym or at home, I never use air conditioning but always keep the windows open.

The best time to run is after 8:00 in the evening or before 7:00 in the morning to avoid inhaling fumes from motor vehicles or industrial plants. Since oxygen intake is increased when running, it is important not to run where you will inhale carbon monoxide or other harmful elements, such as lead and mercury from gasoline, petroleum, or paint, and other chemicals from industry. A large percentage of polluted air is not exhaled, but stored in the body and liable to cause harmful effects such as tension, nervousness, and imbalance of minerals.

Thinking Ahead

In every sense the best medicine is prevention, and this certainly applies to shaping up. On the following pages are a few points on anticipating potential causes of endangered health and well-being.

Jet Lag

High-speed travel across several time zones causes a psychological dislocation of normal body rhythms. Affected are the heart, circulatory system, nervous system, and glands that work together in coordination. As we fly in jet planes at top speed, crossing national and international time boundaries, the close coordination of these vital bodily functions is thrown into confusion. According to studies, the glandular system is the most troubled, since its main controlling agent is the nervous system. In turn, the glands are affected, and their function of secreting hormones to control and coordinate all body activities is disrupted.

To combat jet lag you should prepare yourself before getting on the plane. A heavy training session, running, or a good deal of walking tends to make the body rest better while in flight. Exercising tires your entire system so it undergoes repair conditions while traveling. If you do not exercise, and become restless on the plane, the body builds up tension, causing glands to secrete hormones unnecessarily.

While in flight, drink a good quantity of liquids, since dehydration of body fluids is a prime factor leading to jet lag. I recommend having at least three glasses of noncaffeinated liquids per hour, including beer, small amounts of wine or champagne. Hard alcohol is unadvisable since it accelerates dehydration at double the normal rate. This is not the case with champagne, beer, and wine due to

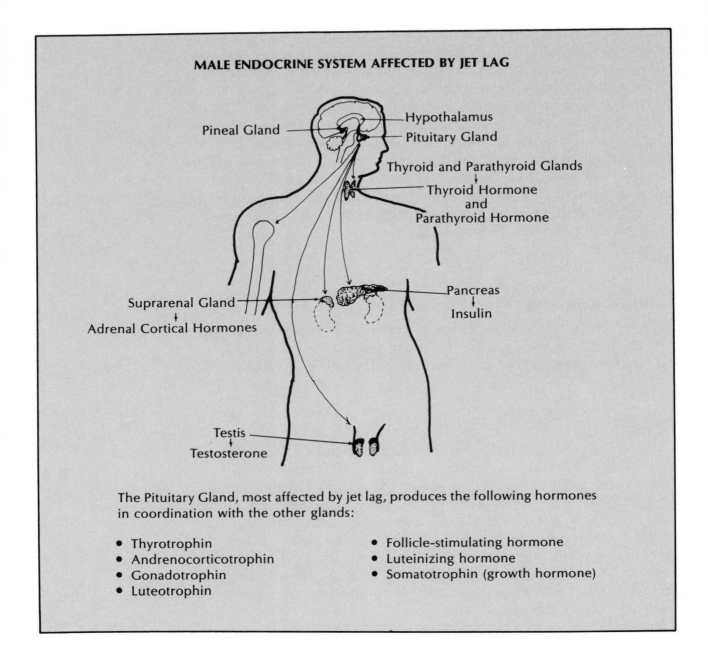

MALE ENDOCRINE SYSTEM AFFECTED BY JET LAG

Pineal Gland

Hypothalamus

Pituitary Gland

Thyroid and Parathyroid Glands
↓
Thyroid Hormone
and
Parathyroid Hormone

Suprarenal Gland
↓
Adrenal Cortical Hormones

Pancreas
↓
Insulin

Testis
↓
Testosterone

The Pituitary Gland, most affected by jet lag, produces the following hormones in coordination with the other glands:

- Thyrotrophin
- Andrenocorticotrophin
- Gonadotrophin
- Luteotrophin

- Follicle-stimulating hormone
- Luteinizing hormone
- Somatotrophin (growth hormone)

their low alcohol content. I also advise eating a lot of fresh fruit rather than the meals provided by the airline. No matter how daintily caterers prepare the food trays, invariably a full meal eaten in flight leads to indigestion. Also, walking around as much as possible on the plane is extremely helpful for the glandular system, helping to maintain its harmony within the network of bodily functions.

After reaching your destination, take a warm shower and then do several stretching exercises, such as the Back Leg Stretch, and abdominal exercises. This miniworkout will help restore the muscular activity of the organs, retarded by the close confines of air travel.

The body seems most affected when flying west to east because this time change is more disruptive to the usual pattern of sleep. Many men traveling to the East Coast try forcing themselves to sleep, making the situation worse through the stress of opposing their ordinary sleep habits. It is far better to stay awake for those extra hours, enjoying some form of entertainment so you will be physically tired and mentally rested at bedtime.

Eye Exercises

Whether or not most people realize it, their eyes have a very limited range of motion as they go through their daily routine of activities. Those working in offices focus mainly on reading material such as columns of figures, computer printouts, correspondence, reports, and articles. Students spend long hours reading books with fine print, and those traveling on the road suffer the stress of glaring sunlight as they keep their eyes fixed on traffic, road signs, and

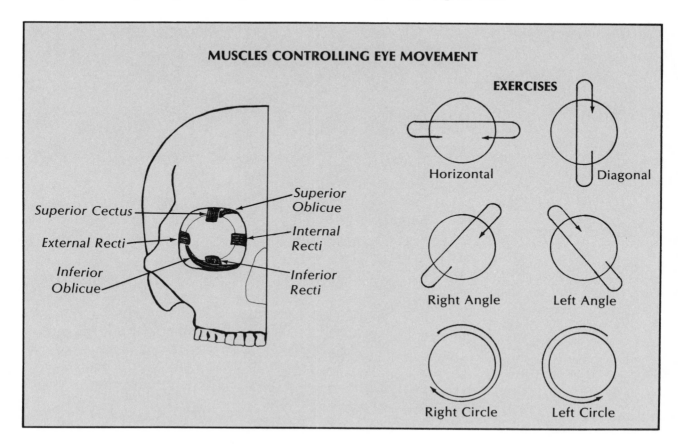

MUSCLES CONTROLLING EYE MOVEMENT

EXERCISES

Superior Cectus

Superior Oblicue

External Recti

Internal Recti

Inferior Oblicue

Inferior Recti

Horizontal

Diagonal

Right Angle

Left Angle

Right Circle

Left Circle

changing traffic lights. Relaxation most often leads to watching television, reading, or playing computer games, none of which gives the eye muscles a full range of motion.

Just as you must keep a muscular balance in exercising the arms or legs, your eyes must be exercised in a variety of ways to prevent atrophy of certain muscles.

The following exercises will help maintain and improve your vision. The series should be done four to six times a week with 20 movements in each direction.

1. Right to left and left to right.
2. Up and down and down and up.
3. Right upper corner to lower left corner.
4. Left upper corner to lower right corner.
5. Rotate to the left.
6. Rotate to the right.

Exercise Glossary

Backhand Stretch

Stand on your toes with arms raised just below shoulder level. Leading with your elbow, snap your arms backward as far as possible.

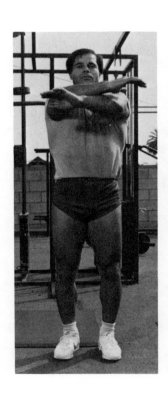
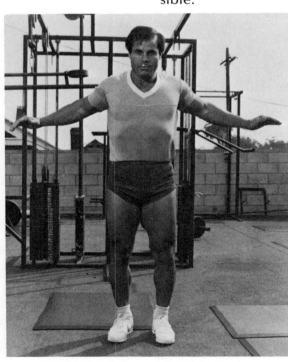

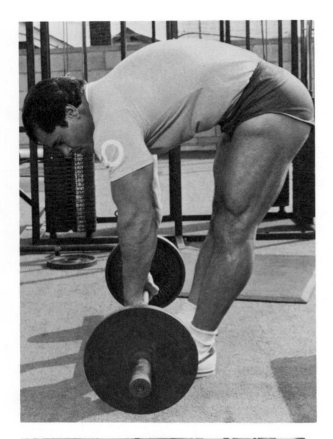

Barbell Row

Bending forward from the waist, grasp the bar with a medium grip, palms held down. Bring the bar to your chest, then lower it. Avoid jerking the bar. Keep the movement smooth and coordinated. **20–60 pounds.**

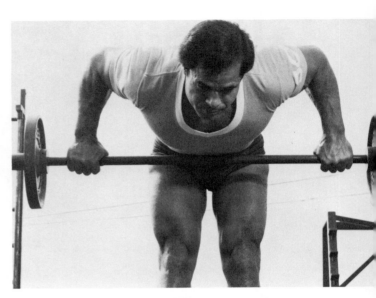

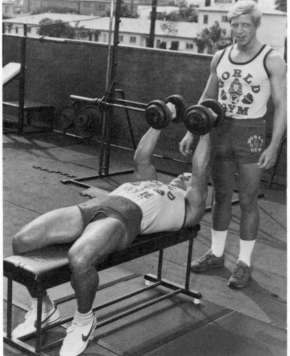

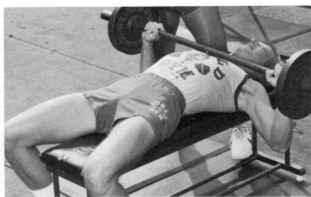

Bench Press

Start by moving the barbell or dumbbells into an upright position over your head. Maintaining a grip 30–40 inches wide, lower the barbell, keeping it level across your chest. Inhale while lowering; exhale on the push-up. Keep your spine straight. **20–60 pounds, or 10–30 pounds per hand.**

Bent-Leg Sit-Up

Lie on your back holding your hands directly over your head. Bend your knees toward your chest, trying to bring them to the elbows. Do not raise your lower back off the floor to avoid straining it.

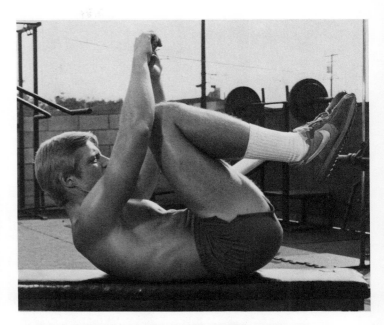

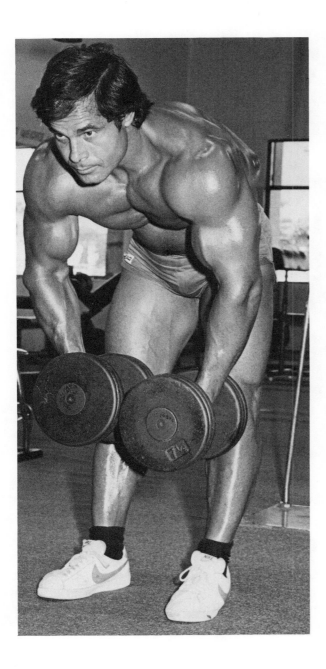

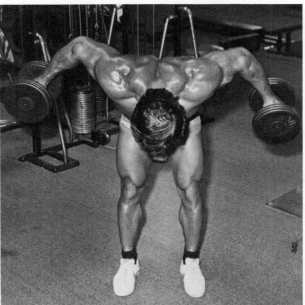

Bent-Over Lateral Raise

Stand grasping a dumbbell in each hand. Keep your feet shoulder width apart. Bend forward from the waist with arms held straight. Pull the elbows up as high as you can, keeping the movement slow and continuous. **5–10 pounds per hand.**

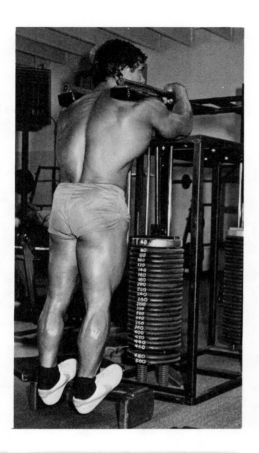

Calf Raise

Stand with the balls of both feet on a block of wood. Holding on to the back of a chair for balance, go up and down on your toes. As shown, you can also use a calf raise machine to add extra weight to the movement.

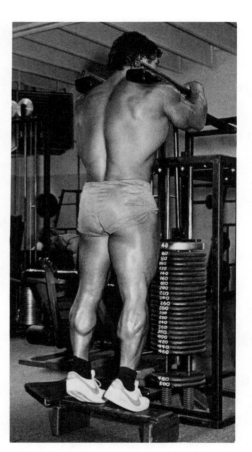

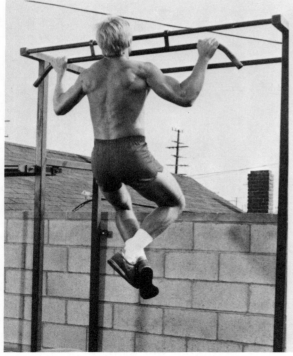

Chin

Grasp the bar with an overgrip, hands set wider than shoulder width. Keeping your back arched, slowly pull your body up to the bar, head in front of, or behind, the bar.

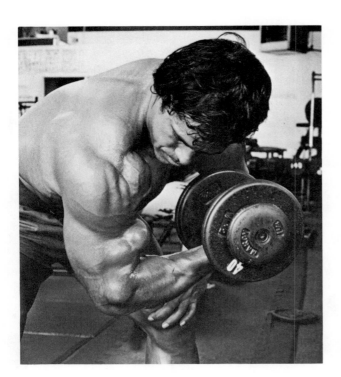

Concentration Curl

Spread your legs and bend your knees. Bend forward and rest your free hand on your knee for some back support. Pick up the dumbbell, keeping your arm vertical and curl as correctly as possible.

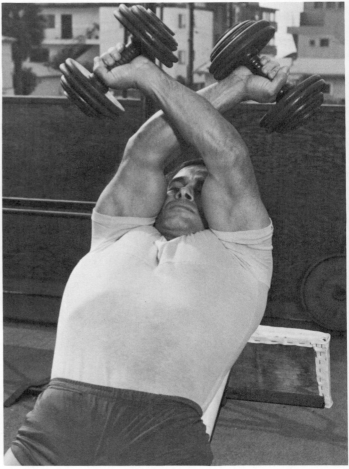

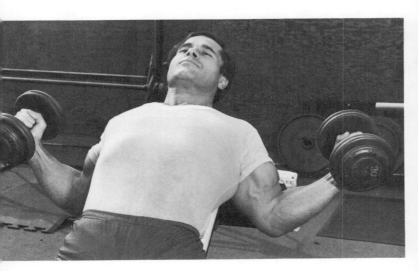

Cross Flye

Lie on your back on the floor or a small bench, holding a dumbbell in each hand. Starting with the arms outstretched to both sides, raise both arms straight up and cross them. Control the movement, advancing each arm equally. **5–10 pounds per hand.**

Crunch Sit-Up

Lie on your back on the floor with your legs on top of a bench or chair. Keep the knees bent. Clasping your hands over your chest, raise the upper body close to your knees.

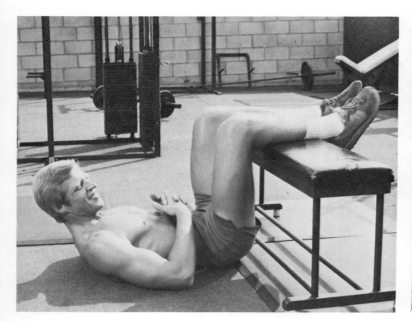

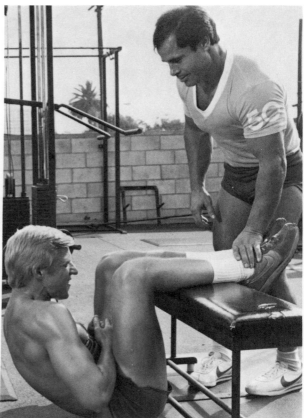

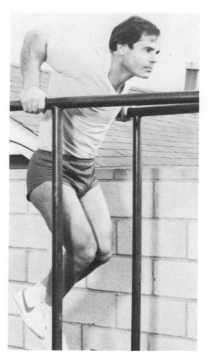

Dip

Use either parallel bars or chairs, holding on with a tight grip. Look forward throughout the exercise. Inhale going down as low as possible; exhale on raising yourself with the force of the chest, shoulders, and arms.

Donkey Kick

Get on your hands and knees, bending the elbows slightly for leverage. Keeping one leg straight, raise it up as high behind you as possible, and then down again while contracting the buttocks.

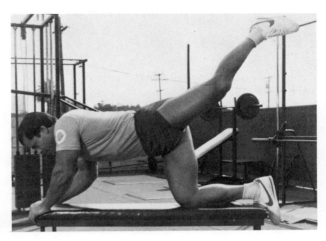

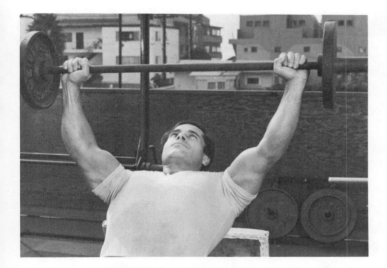

Incline Bench Raise (Press)

On an incline bench, start with the bar held over the eyes. Inhaling deeply, lower the bar to just below your neck. Exhale, pushing the bar back to the starting position. **20–60 pounds.**

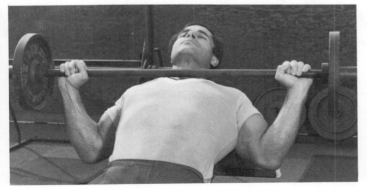

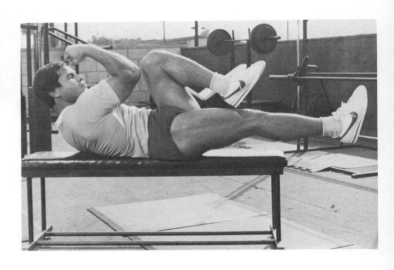

Knee to Elbow

Lie on your back on the floor with both hands clasped behind your head. Bending one leg at a time, and raising the neck and head from the floor, bring the opposite knee and elbow together.

Lateral Raise

Holding a dumbbell in each hand, stand with feet 12 inches apart. Bend the elbows slightly and raise the dumbbells a little higher than shoulder level. **5–10 pounds per hand.**

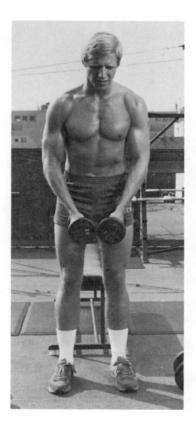 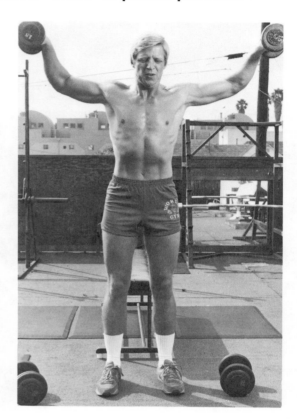

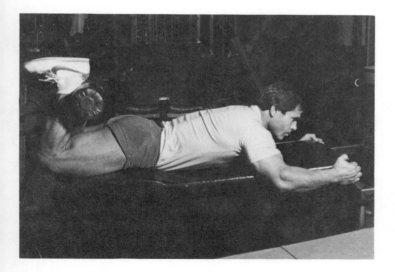

Leg Curl

Lie on your stomach on a bench, holding on to the bench edge to stabilize your body. Raise your chest off the bench but keep your hips in place. Place the weight across your ankles. Keeping the movement fluid, straighten your legs completely on the way down and try to touch your thighs on the way up. **10–30 pounds.**

Leg Extension

Sit on a bench or sturdy chair. Place your hands on your hips or hold on to the bench. Placing the weight on your ankles, extend legs straight on the way up, then bend them on the way down. **10–30 pounds.**

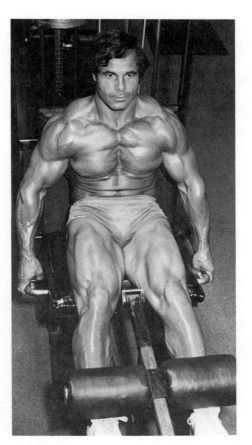

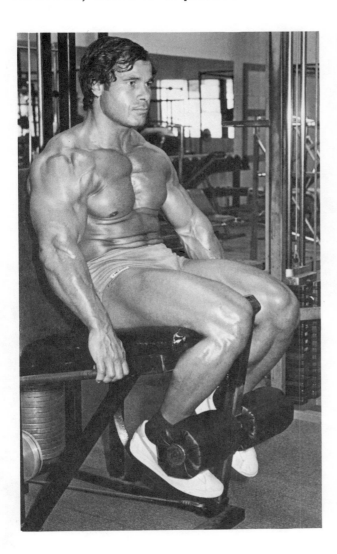

Leg Raise

Lie on your back on the floor or a bench. Keep your hands straight down or grip the bench behind your head. Holding the knees flexed and the toes pointed, raise both legs straight up together. Keep your hips on the bench.

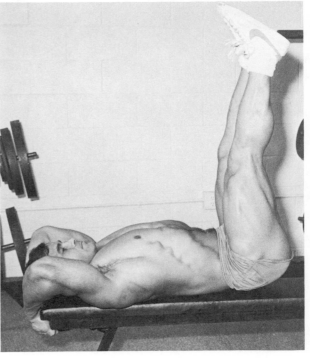

Lunge

Stand holding a book or weight in each hand. Step forward with the left foot as far as possible, lowering the body until your right knee almost touches the floor. Step back and repeat the lunge, starting with the right foot. **5–10 pounds per hand.**

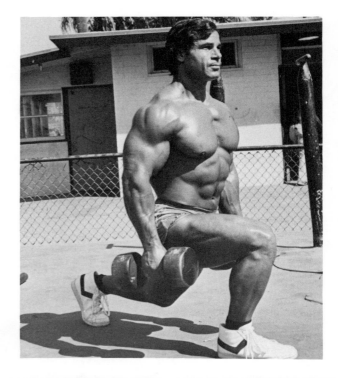

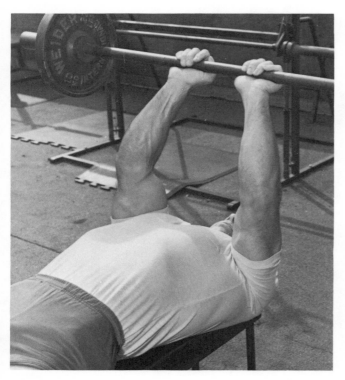

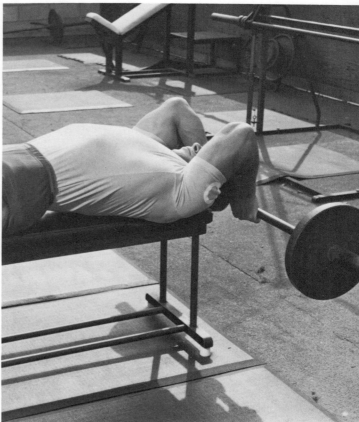

Lying Barbell Triceps Extension

Hold a barbell with your elbows facing up. Lower the bar to your forehead, then raise it again for a complete extension without moving your elbows. **20–60 pounds.**

One-Arm Rowing

Stand with your legs apart and your upper body parallel to the floor. Start with the dumbbell held just above the floor between your legs. Pull the dumbbell up, touching the side of the pectoral muscle, then lower it for a complete stretch. Do the exercise at a rapid pace. **10–30 pounds.**

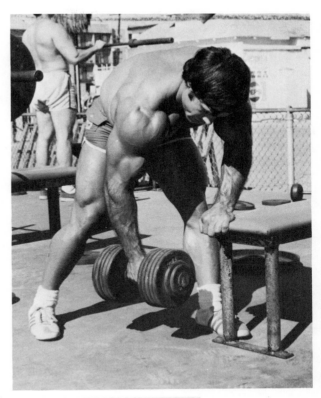

Preacher Bench Curl

Grasp a barbell with hands held 10–14 inches apart. Holding your palms face up, curl the barbell up to your chin, then extend your arms. Keep your elbows 10–14 inches apart. **10–30 pounds.**

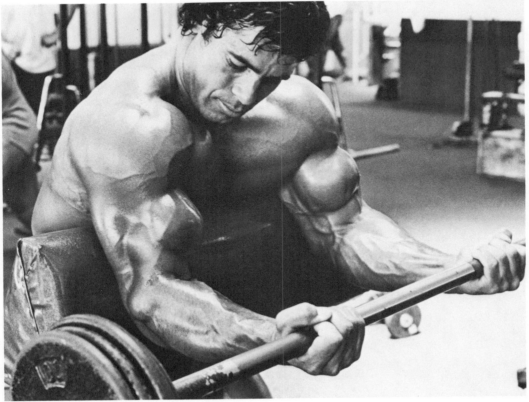

Press behind Neck

While standing or sitting, hold the bar with a medium-wide grip. Inhale while lowering the bar to the base of your neck, then quickly press it overhead while exhaling. Keep your back straight, preferably braced, and perform the reps without pausing. **20–60 pounds.**

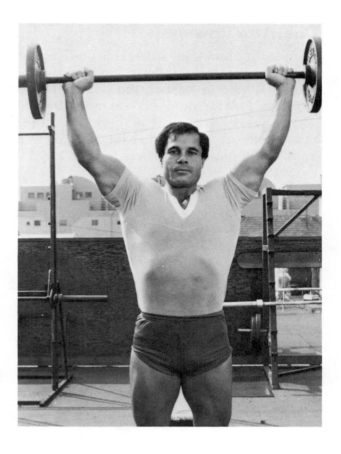

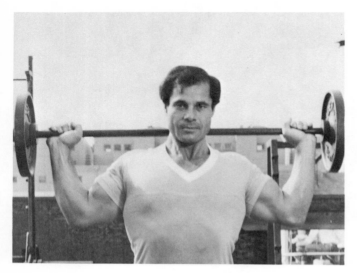

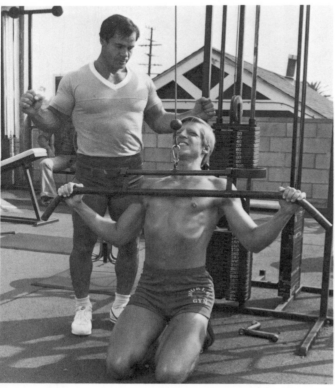

Pulldown

Kneel on the floor. Take the weight bar behind your neck or in front and pull it down as far as possible. Raise it and pull it down again, exhaling as you pull down. **20–60 pounds.**

Pullover

Lie on your back on a bench or across a chair, holding dumbbells or a barbell overhead with slightly bent arms. When using a barbell, grip it no wider than your shoulders. Slowly lower the weight behind your head, inhaling as you lower it. Exhale as you return to the starting position. Here a good stretch is important. **10–30 pounds, total.**

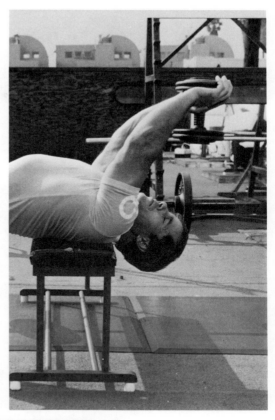

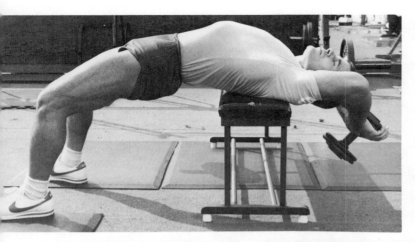

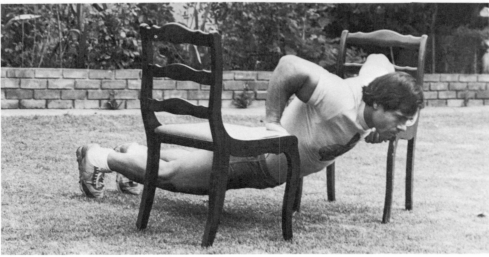

Push-Up Using Chairs

Place two chairs about 24 inches apart. Position body so each hand is on a chair and torso angles between the chairs. Push the entire body weight slowly up and down, trying for a complete range of motion.

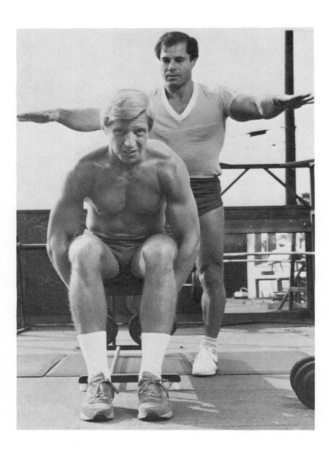

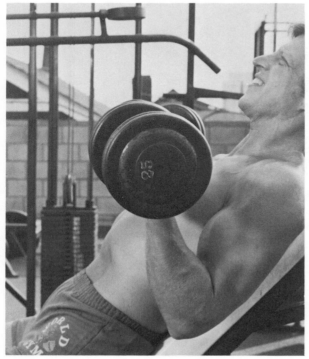

Seated Bent-Over Lateral Raise

Sit on the edge of a chair with your knees slightly bent. Start with your upper body bent over 30–40 degrees. Keeping your elbows bent, lift the dumbbells laterally as high as you can. **5–15 pounds per hand.**

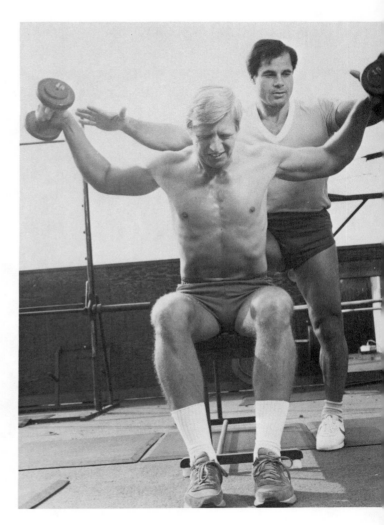

Seated Dumbbell Curl

Sit on a chair, holding a dumbbell in each hand. Curl the dumbbells up toward your shoulder, then down again, turning your wrists outward as you curl. **5–15 pounds per hand.**

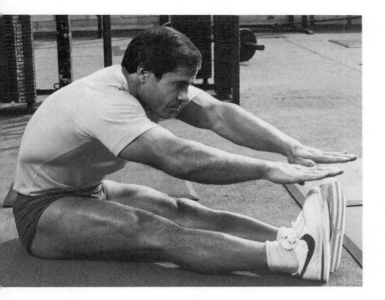

Seated Hamstring Stretch

Sit on the floor with legs straight out and together, toes curved toward the upper body. Slowly reach forward as far as you can without bending the knees. Hold the tips of your toes for 5–10 seconds. Return slowly to the starting position.

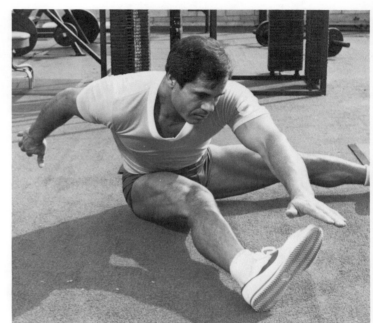

Seated Stretch

Sit on the floor with your legs spread wide and knees held straight. Stretch the right hand to the left foot and then the left hand to the right foot, alternating between them at a fast pace.

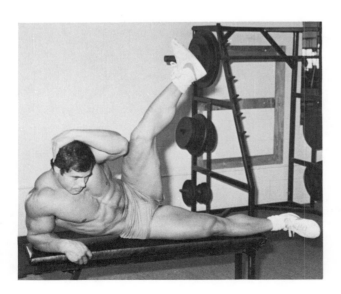

Side Leg Raise

Lie on one side, supported by your elbow. Keep the upper leg straight, bending the other for a base of support. Raise and lower the upper arm and leg at the same time.

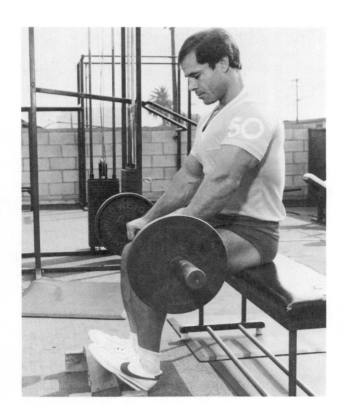

Sitting Calf Raise

If you do not have access to a calf machine, use a barbell. Sit on a bench and use a calf block. Place the bar on top of your thighs and hold it with your hands while raising and lowering your feet as far as possible. **30–70 pounds.**

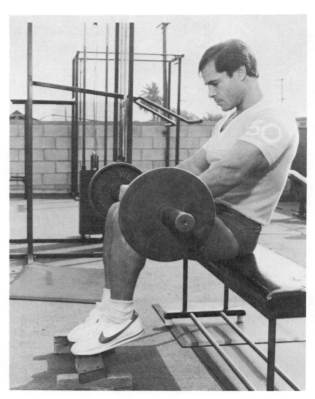

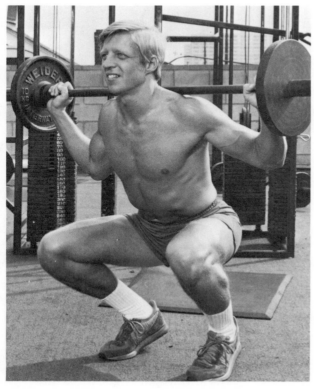

Squat

Stand with your heels on a block of wood or telephone book two inches high. Slowly bend into a full squat, keeping control of the movement. Slowly stand.

Squat with Bar on Shoulders

Stand with heels 12 inches apart on a wood block two inches high. Looking straight ahead will help control the movement. Work with the barbell on your shoulders, lowering the body slowly into a full squat. Slowly stand. **20–60 pounds.**

Standing Hamstring Stretch

Stand with one foot on the edge of a chair, the heel pointing downward. Keeping both legs straight, reach forward until you feel a good stretch along the back of your leg. Hold a moment, keeping the spine as straight as possible to promote increased motion in the lower back. Perform slowly without forcing the stretch.

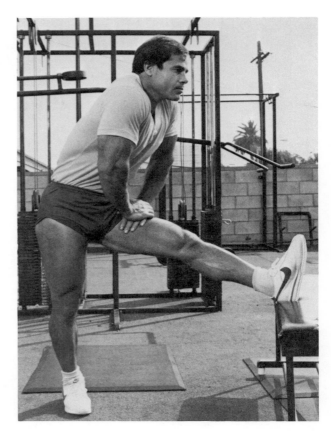

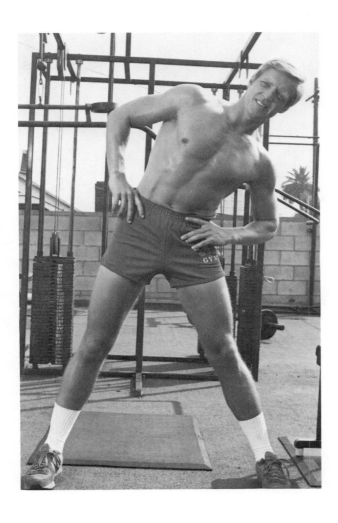

Standing Side Bend

Stand with hands on hips, feet spread far apart. Alternate bending slowly from right to left, each time holding the position for a moment.

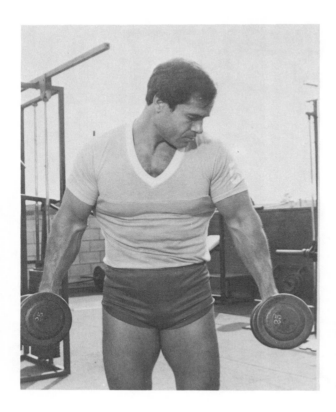

Standing Wrist Curl

Standing erect, hold a dumbbell in each hand with the palms held inward. Move your hands outward and feel both sides of the forearm muscles moving. **5–15 pounds per hand.**

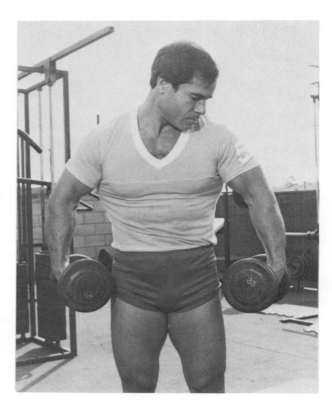

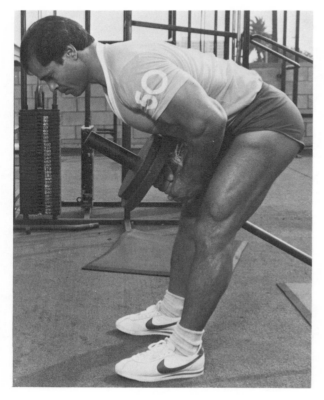

T-Bar Rowing

Stand with feet approximately 15 inches apart. Bend from the waist and keep your knees slightly bent. Grab one end of a T-bar or barbell and pull it toward your stomach in a smooth movement. Lower to full extension. Do not jerk the bar. **20–50 pounds.**

Triceps Pushdown

Use a close grip and bend forward slightly. Push the bar down until your arms are straight. Exhale when pushing down and do all the reps in one continuous motion. **20–60 pounds.**

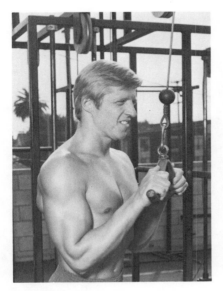

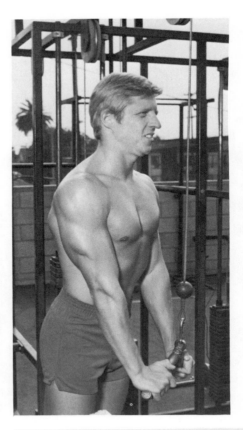

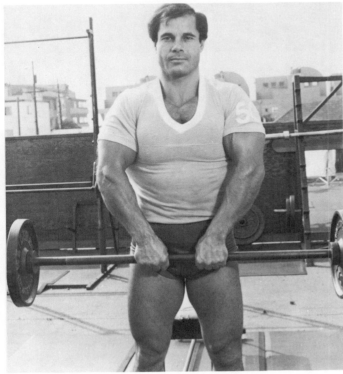

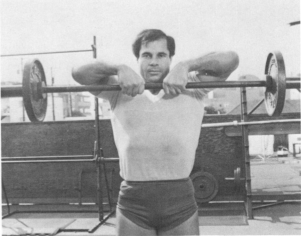

Upright Rowing

Use an overhand grip, picking up the barbell with hands held six inches apart. Pull the bar up to your chin and lower it again to thigh level. Exhale while pulling up; inhale while lowering the barbell. **20–40 pounds.**

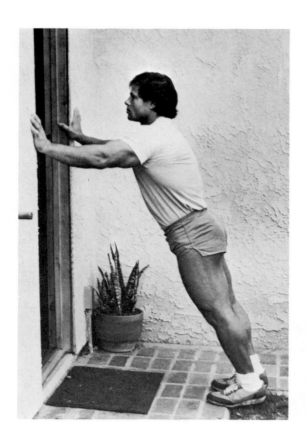

Wall Push-Up

Standing three or four feet from the corner of a room, place one hand on each wall at shoulder height. Hold the body and stomach muscles rigid as you slowly move forward and touch your chin to the corner of the wall. Slowly return to the starting position.

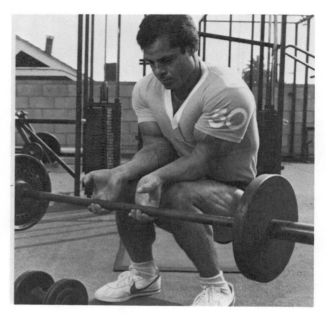

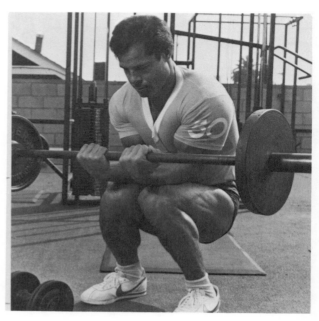

Wrist Curl

Start with your arms supported by a bench or other flat surface such as a stool. Keep the elbows still and straight. Curl the wrists upward. **20–40 pounds.**

Index